Caring for People

A Lifespan Approach

Judy Richards

Stanley Thornes (Publishers) Ltd

Text © Judy Richards 1999
Original line illustrations © Stanley Thornes Publishers Ltd

First published 1999 by
Stanley Thornes Publishers Ltd
Ellenborough House
Wellington Street
Cheltenham
GL50 1YW
UK

ISBN 0 7487 3900 9

99 00 01 02 03 / 10 9 8 7 6 5 4 3 2 1

Illustrations by Oxford Designers and Illustrators and Jean de Lemos, Graham-Cameron Illustrations
Typeset by Northern Phototypesetting Company Ltd, Bolton
Printed and bound in Great Britain by Redwood Books, Trowbridge, Wiltshire

Contents

Acknowledgements

The author and publishers would like to thank the following organisations for permission to reproduce material: the British Association of Social Workers and the United Kingdom Central Council for Nursing, Midwifery and Health Visiting.

Every effort has been made to contact copyright holders and we apologise if any have been overlooked.

I would also like to thank Doreen Rowe for her excellent typing support; Peter Sharples, Principal, colleagues and students of Coulsdon College, Surrey; my mother, Mrs Nansi Thomas, her friends and care workers at Castle View Rest Home, Llawhaden, Pembrokeshire, West Wales; my colleague Gill Taylor who was my first 'official' reader; and my supportive friends Esther, Marg and André.

Further acknowledgements

My mother died peacefully on 27 May 1999 before this book was published. I would like to thank Ward 12, Withybush Hospital, Haverfordwest, Pembrokeshire for their exceptional nursing care, and Bethany Free Church for their spiritual care and support.

Judy Richards

Dedication

To Jeff, Jessica, Helen and Nan

Introduction

Caring for People: A Lifespan Approach aims to provide readers with the basic introductory knowledge and understanding required for effective care work. The book is divided into two parts:

- Part 1 covers the key concepts, values and skills that all care workers should be aware of and understand. It is written in a general way so that what the reader learns can be applied in a variety of different care settings. It also brings into sharper focus the need for carers to *care* for themselves and for others.
- Part 2 applies these key concepts to work with different client groups across the lifespan. The client groups covered are: babies, children, adolescents and teenagers, adults and older people. Each client group is covered in a separate chapter, which provides relevant information on growth and development issues, health and social care needs and the different approaches used in care work with members of the specified client group.

Key words and phrases are emboldened in the text, listed in *Key Terms* at the end of each chapter and defined in the Glossary on pages 167–73.

It is possible to use the book as a 'continuous read' as the chapters are designed to build on each other in developing and explaining key ideas and approaches to caring for people. Alternatively, if you have a particular interest in a topic, or client group, the chapters can be used in a separate 'stand alone' way.

PART 1

KEY CONCEPTS OF CARING

Part 1 looks at some of the key aspects with regard to caring. The chapters are:

1 ▷ *An introduction to caring*

2 ▷ *Qualities and skills for caring*

3 ▷ *Values for caring*

4 ▷ *Holistic care*

5 ▷ *Aspects of care*

Following a brief introduction to caring, the qualities and skills necessary to enhance the caring process are explored. Integrated into this are the different values involved in caring. The chapter on holistic care identifies the need to care for the whole person. While the chapter on aspects of care looks closely at specific issues including assessment, care planning and caring for the carer.

An introduction to caring

PREVIEW

This chapter is an introduction to some of the basic ideas about caring and care work. The key topics covered in the chapter are:
- The nature of caring
- Reasons for choosing caring as a career
- Carers and care services
- The care relationship.

Care is provided by a range of people and organisations, the choice of which is dependent on the type of care required to meet the needs of the individual concerned. A person who takes on the role of carer therefore requires a variety of skills to ensure that those needs are met. It is important to identify the nature of caring and to explore the different aspects which contribute to the role of carer.

THE NATURE OF CARING

Thinking about the nature of caring raises the questions, 'What is caring?' and 'What does caring for others really mean?' If you have enrolled on a Health and Social Care course, you will probably have some ideas about this already. It is important to identify the different issues which relate to caring and to think hard about what is involved in caring.

'Caring' is a word that has different meanings. It is used to describe an individual's:

- *personal qualities* – people may talk about someone as being 'a caring person' or they may say 'that person was really caring towards me'. These comments refer to caring as being a personal quality or feature of that person's personality. People who are attracted to care work will often say that they are 'a caring person' and that they have 'caring qualities', such as patience, kindness and understanding

- *behaviour* – people may be able to perform an act of kindness or may go out of their way to carry out a practical task with a smile. This is viewed as caring behaviour.

However, in the caring profession, the term 'caring' carries much more meaning than just being kind or performing an act of kindness. Though certainly, carers and care workers need to draw on such qualities in themselves in order to do their job.

In the context of care work, caring can be defined as giving support to individuals who:

- need help with daily living activities, for example, making a cup of tea, helping them to the bathroom, helping with the housework, or just calling in for a chat and to check they are alright
- have more complex health-related needs, which require more skilled help, such as using a hoist to have a bath, recording and monitoring the heart beat using a cardiograph.

While a caring personality will greatly assist a person in providing such care, carers also need to have a clear understanding of the individual needs of clients. This involves the ability to:

- communicate effectively with people
- have a basic understanding of the variety of methods that can be used to help and support people.

These abilities are developed through a fundamental understanding of the theory and practice of caring which are covered in the following chapters of Part 1.

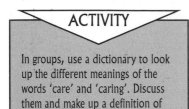

ACTIVITY

In groups, use a dictionary to look up the different meanings of the words 'care' and 'caring'. Discuss them and make up a definition of 'caring' in the context of the caring professions.

CASE STUDY

Mary

Mary is a GNVQ Health and Social Care student who is starting work experience. Her placement is at Cherry Trees Residential Home for the Elderly. Her college tutor has agreed with the home that Mary will spend three weeks working with the clients on a daily basis. Mary is very anxious about her first day, as she has no experience of working with older people. Her grandparents are still only in their early sixties, are reasonably active and have many interests.

1 What are the issues which face Mary in this placement?

2 What advice would you give Mary about her placement?

3 What support should be given to Mary during her placement?

REASONS FOR CHOOSING CARING AS A CAREER

'Why choose caring as a career?' is a question that many people ask those who enter the caring field. People are attracted to a career in care work for a variety of different reasons. For example, they may have:

- *previous experience of caring for others*, for example, baby-sitting, caring for an older relative, supporting a friend who has been involved in a car accident, sitting with a neighbour who is going through a bereavement
- *previous experience of being cared for*, for example, a short stay in hospital following treatment, support from a friend during a difficult period
- *observed positive care in action, which motivates them towards the caring profession and provides them with a role model*, for example, visiting a relative in hospital and observing nurses, taking a younger brother or sister to nursery and observing the nursery workers or visiting an older relative in a residential home and observing the caring attitude of the care assistants.

There are many different reasons why individuals become involved in caring for other people. A desire to help and support others, accompanied by a caring personality or temperament are considered to be important starting points in the process of caring for others. But, while these aspects are important, it is also essential to remember that caring for others can be demanding and stressful. Stress is discussed in Chapter 5.

Carers and care workers are involved in providing a range of different care services, requiring various skills to meet the individual needs of the clients being cared for.

CARERS AND CARE SERVICES

Care can basically be described as either **formal care** or **informal care**.

- *Formal care* is provided by professional, employed carers who look after and support individuals in formal care settings, for example, registered general nurses, health care assistants, district nurses, health visitors.
- *Informal care* is provided by relatives, friends, volunteers or neighbours who give support to an individual, usually in that person's home, without pay. Informal care can range from caring for an older parent and supporting all their daily needs to regularly visiting a disabled person at home for a chat, checking that all is well and having a cup of tea with them.

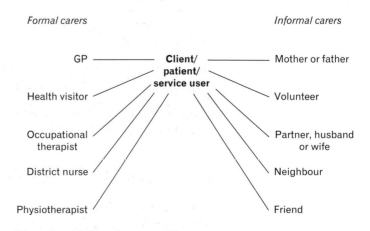

Examples of formal and informal care providers

Carers and care workers

In this book, two different terms refer to people who provide care.

- *Care worker* is used to refer to an individual who is employed to provide care for other people, i.e. a *formal* carer. This includes all types of paid professional care workers, for example, those care workers who are employed in residential homes, hospitals, day nurseries and clients' homes.

- *Carer* is used to refer to people who provide care on an *informal*, voluntary and unpaid basis, for example, close relatives, such as the person's own children or parents, or their friends or neighbours. Carers often take on considerable responsibilities when providing care for another person. In doing so, they may or may not get help and support from a care worker. Voluntary carers are usually those people who offer their services to care charities or voluntary organisations such as the Women's Royal Voluntary Service (WRVS) or Help the Aged.

Types of care

The types of care that a carer or care worker provides cover a range of tasks. Parker and Lawton (1994) provide the following task-focused typology of activities that can be called caring:

- *help with personal care* such as washing, toileting, etc.
- *help with paper work or financial matters* such as keeping up-to-date with letters, paying bills, applying for benefit
- *practical help*, such as shopping, housework, gardening
- *keeping the helped person company* including talking, chatting, joining in leisure activities, watching television
- *taking the helped person out* by, for example, arranging trips and taking them on outings
- *giving medicines*, such as tablets and injections
- *keeping an eye on the helped person* by, for example, calling in on them at home and checking that they have not had a fall or been taken ill.

The people receiving care

People who are at the receiving end of the care process are referred to as:

- *clients* – generally by health and social care providers, for example, in residential homes or day care, or
- *patients* – generally by hospital staff and other health-care providers, or
- *service users* – generally by social care providers, such as the staff of drop-in centres.

In this book, *client* is used for convenience, but its use implies *patients* and *service users* too.

Organisational categories of care

Many health and social care organisations, such as NHS Trust hospitals and local authority social services departments, arrange their caring services into the following organisational categories:

- *acute health care services* – medical and surgical treatments and follow-up care, for example emergency health services, district general hospitals, nursing homes
- *continuing care services* – continuous services, which are provided to meet the ongoing, different health and social care needs of individuals with chronic (long-term) conditions, for example care services for older people, home-help services providing home carers
- *social care services* – care services which support the physical, intellectual, emotional, social and cultural needs of the individual, for example, residential care, day care
- *priority services* – emergency or immediate care services, for example, ambulance and paramedic services.

Direct and indirect care

As has been seen, caring is maintained by different carers and care workers in a range of settings and services. Carers and care workers are usually involved in *direct care*, which basically means working *with* clients and carrying out the different caring tasks.

However, there is a large number of *indirect carers* who support the caring services, without any contact with a client, for example, laboratory technicians and catering staff.

Levels of formal care

There are three levels of formal care provided by professional care workers.

- *Primary care* is given at the first stage of the care or treatment process. This includes school health services, home caring and nursing services, GP services.
- *Secondary care* is health and care which is referred on from primary care. This includes acute hospital services, such as the local general hospital or hospital trust
- *Tertiary care* is offered through specialised hospital services. This includes specialist hospital treatment, such as at the Royal Marsden NHS Trust which specialises in cancer care.

These levels of care are closely associated with the different care settings described below.

Care settings

Care settings are the different contexts (places) in which caring takes place. They may operate on a short-term basis, i.e. a few hours a day, and offer a range of services, such as a chiropodist and a hairdresser, or they may operate on a long-term basis with full 24-hour care.

ACTIVITY

a) In pairs, make a list of the different primary care, secondary care and tertiary care providers in your local area.

b) Join with a larger group and share information.

Examples of care settings are as follows.

- *Domiciliary care* This is carried out in the client's home. Informal carers will usually include relatives, friends, neighbours. Formal carers who come into domiciliary settings are usually nurses, home helps or home carers, care assistants and GPs.

- *Day care* This is carried out in a day centre or day hospital. Informal carers may be volunteers. Formal carers are usually care managers, care assistants, plus support staff such as cleaners, cooks and building maintenance workers.

- *Residential care* This is carried out in nursing and residential homes, hostels, long-stay hospitals and community-based homes. Informal carers may be volunteers, relatives or friends of the people receiving care. Formal carers are usually care managers, care assistants, plus support staff such as cleaners, cooks, building maintenance workers

- *Hospital care* This usually involves complex medical or surgical interventions or an emergency admission. For example, surgery is nearly always carried out in a hospital. Formal carers are doctors, nurses, health-care assistants. Informal carers are family, friends, neighbours, volunteer helpers.

An important role of the carer or care worker is to ensure that the care setting is safe, secure, comfortable and a pleasant place to live or stay.

CASE STUDY

Brian

Brian is an active 80-year-old widower who lives in a small cottage in a country village. He has no family living nearby. His younger brother, who is 65, lives 100 miles away. His neighbour Joan pops in twice a week to help with housework and the shopping. One day Brian slips in the garden and twists his ankle. His GP visits and tells him he should rest the ankle for at least three weeks. Brian has a problem since he knows Joan works part-time and has a husband and three children to look after. Brian needs support.

1 What types of care did Brian experience before his accident?

2 What types of care does he need now? Are there different levels of care involved?

3 How would you organise his care? What recommendations would you make to Brian?

4 Who will be his formal and informal carers?

THE CARE RELATIONSHIP

Carers and care workers provide a service for clients, patients and service users. In doing so, they will build up a professional **care relationship**. This is the relationship which is built up between a carer or care worker and a client.

The care relationship is the cornerstone of the whole caring process. In the caring context, carers and care workers, clients, patients and service users have various ideas about what the relationship between them and the person being helped should be like. Like any other relationship, care relationships can run into difficulties at times and, when problems can't be overcome, can fail. Some of the problems which can occur are identified in Chapter 5. Strategies to resolve these problems are also addressed.

In this section, we will consider the factors that influence the development of care relationships,

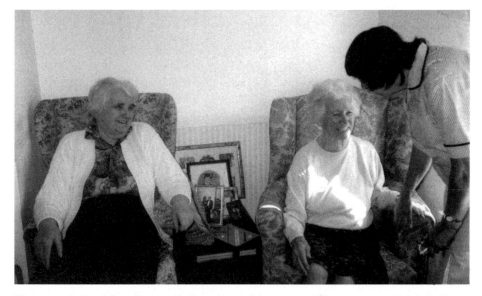

The care relationship – the carer is listening, talking and building a rapport with her clients

Factors influencing effective care relationships

A number of factors determine how effective the caring process is and how well a care relationship can be built up. These factors include:

- *time* – How much time does the carer spend caring – is it a shift of 12 hours, 3 or 4 times a week, a 1-hour visit a week or 24 hours daily?

- *the care setting* – Is there appropriate equipment, resources and space? Is the environment healthy and safe?

- *skills and expertise* – Is the carer trained to manage the different caring tasks and activities? Have they the necessary knowledge to maintain the care process?

- *support* – Is relevant and appropriate support available for the carer? Is there a line of support, for example, line managers, or a network of support, for example, voluntary groups?

- *needs* – Are the needs of the carers and those being helped clearly identified?

An effective, mutually beneficial care relationship is very important as it makes the task of assessing and meeting the needs of the client far easier.

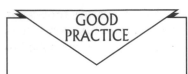

GOOD PRACTICE

These guidelines will support carers and care workers who are embarking on a career in caring. By bearing these points in mind, carers can develop positive, supportive caring relationships. Although they appear to be basic requirements for all jobs, they are particularly important features of caring and form the basis of the care relationship.

- Punctuality – always turn up at the agreed time.
- Attendance – turn up on agreed days, shifts, visiting times. If you are unable to attend, give the appropriate people adequate notice.
- Get to know your client – be polite, spend time introducing yourself, listening to the client, sharing news, etc.
- Find your way around the care setting – look round, find emergency exits, check the setting with regard to health and safety, i.e. carry out a risk assessment.
- Emergency contact – make sure that you know who to call if necessary.
- Information – make sure you read the client's case notes, or have been adequately informed through a reporting procedure so that you:
  - can carry out the requirements of the care plan, for example, you may need to change a catheter bag. Do you know what it is? Have you done it before?
  - can use any specialised equipment which is necessary for the client
  - know about the disorder, disease or dysfunction of the client. This will save you having to ask too many questions which may make the client feel uneasy. Let them volunteer information about their condition
  - can find out the procedures with regard to confidentiality,

The care relationship is not just based on initial impressions, it develops gradually over a period of time. However, those initial impressions *can* give the client a positive or negative idea about a carer. So the basic requirements listed here under *Good Practice* are necessary for a positive start to the care relationship.

CASE STUDY

Eddie

Eddie is 3 years old and lives with his mother in a reception centre for homeless families. They are waiting to be rehoused and therefore Eddie does not attend any local pre-school or early years centre. The local authority has arranged for him to be visited by a play worker. Her name is Mavis and she visits Eddie every week bringing toys and games and different activities for them to do together. Eddie really looks forward to Mavis' weekly visits and his mother enjoys having another adult to talk to. One day, Mavis does not turn up, and she does not let the family know. Eddie is very upset and angry and cries when she does not appear. The next week Mavis turns up as usual and Eddie will not talk to her.

1 What are the issues involved in this case study?

2 What has Mavis done to jeopardise the care relationship?

3 Make suggestions as to how this care relationship can be restored.

Establishing a long-term care relationship is a continual process for all those involved. The carer or care worker should also take into account their working relationship with other carers and care managers, as well as with the client, their family and friends.

There are a number of key questions which a carer and care worker may want to ask themselves as they reflect on their care practice. These are (Clarke, Sachs and Ford, 1995):

- What are the values upon which I am establishing this relationship?
- How do I personally feel about this client?
- Are there any conflicts between my values and how I feel?
- What am I communicating to this client, both verbally and non-verbally?
- Am I and the client considered equal partners in the relationship?
- Am I clear about what the outcome of this relationship is to be?
- To what extent does this relationship require an emotional component, and how will I manage it?
- How long is this relationship likely to last?

ACTIVITY

In small groups discuss the questions above. Why do you think these questions are important in establishing long-term care relationships?

challenging behaviour, risk assessment and record-keeping.

- Be prepared to learn from the client. Often the client is more experienced in working with carers, and knows about his/her needs, and how they can be met.
- Use a new situation as an opportunity for the client to explain different ways of carrying out tasks. This gives the client a sense that they are part of the process and builds trust and respect. However, remember to check any changes with other carers and the care manager.

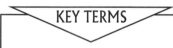

KEY TERMS

You need to know the meaning of the following words and phrases. Go back through the chapter to make sure that you understand them.

acute health care services
care relationship
continuing care services
day care
domiciliary care
formal care
hospital care
informal care
primary care
priority services
residential care
secondary care
social care services
tertiary care

As part of his research, the psychologist Biestek (1992) suggests that carers and care workers need to think carefully about a number of key elements in the care relationship. These mainly relate to clients, but could be applied to colleagues and managers. These elements include:

- *sensitivity* – the care worker must demonstrate sensitivity to the client's feelings at all times. This is not just understanding on the part of the care worker, but includes *demonstrating* the use of effective communication skills
- *understanding* – the special kind of understanding that is typical of the caring relationship is that which is wholly in relation to the client – who they are and what difficulties they may be facing
- *response to the client* – while there may be many practical tasks involved in caring for the client, response must always incorporate feelings. These feelings may be communicated either verbally or non-verbally. The response the care worker makes to the client should communicate an acceptance of that client (see page 18).

KEY POINT

The care relationship is very important – it is a means whereby carer and client can build up a mutually beneficial relationship within which the needs of the client can be adequately assessed and met. It also ensures that effective ways of working with others are addressed.

The qualities and skills necessary to build up an effective care relationship (caring qualities, empathy, self-awareness and communication skills) are discussed further in Chapter 2.

Whether you are already pursuing a career in caring or just entering the caring profession, you will learn that 'acts of kindness which support a person' will develop to include the ability to:

- assess the individual needs of the client, including the setting up of care plans (discussed in Chapter 5)
- protect the rights and choices of clients and support the care value base (discussed in Chapter 3)
- use different methods of treatment and therapy
- work with different professionals within the health and social care field.

Finally, it should be said that becoming a carer and care-giver involves facing many difficult issues, whether you are an informal carer looking after close relatives or friends or a formal carer tending clients and patients in a care setting, such as a hospital ward or a residential home.

Qualities and skills for caring

PREVIEW

People involved in caring for others tend to possess, and are able to use, a number of personal qualities and basic skills in their care relationships. Throughout the chapter we will explore the nature of these key qualities and skills. The key topics covered in this chapter are:

- Caring qualities
- Empathy
- Self-awareness
- Communication skills.

The qualities and skills necessary to build a positive care relationship involve a number of issues which arise in the specific context of the care process. It has been recognised, in Chapter 1, that personal qualities linked with appropriate behaviour are basic requirements in care practice. However, it is important to identify the personal qualities specifically appropriate to the caring profession.

CARING QUALITIES

When an individual works as a carer they need to be able to bring certain qualities into the care relationships that they develop with their clients. These caring qualities, such as kindness, patience and compassion, are often evident in a carer's behaviour towards a client, patient or service user, and are obviously important features of care relationships.

The five Cs of caring

Simone Roach, a Canadian nurse and writer, believes that 'caring embodies certain qualities and specific characteristics'. She calls these the **five Cs of caring** (Roach, 1987). Each of the five Cs relates to a personal quality that

ACTIVITY

In small groups:

a) Discuss, and make a list of, the key qualities that you feel you can make use of in a care relationship.

b) If you were drawing up a job description for a person to look after you, what personal qualities would you list as:
  - essential
  - desirable.

an individual ought to bring to their care relationsh

- compassion
- conscience
- commitment
- confidence
- competence.

Compassion

Compassion is a key quality that 'involves more than acts of kindness, it includes the feelings of the carer, the ability to "get alongside" the individual who is suffering' (Tschudin, 1995). H.J. Nouwen, a researcher and writer, also mentions compassion as being an important quality for caring. She defines it as follows:

'Compassion asks us to go where it hurts, to enter a place of pain, to share in brokenness, fear, confusion and anguish. Compassion challenges us to cry out to those who are in misery, mourn with those who are in tears. Compassion requires us to be weak with the weak, vulnerable with the vulnerable and powerless with the powerless. Compassion means full immersion in the condition of being human' (Nouwen *et al.*, 1982).

This definition identifies and explores the emotional depth with which the carer is able to care. Many caring skills can be learnt, but compassion is perhaps a quality that comes out of the experience of having been hurt oneself and having been shown compassion by another person. Verena Tschudin, a nurse and writer, makes the point that 'we do not respond with compassion out of a sense of duty but out of solidarity' (Tschudin, 1995).

Compassion may be developed in a carer who has faced a similar painful incident in their lives. They are reminded of the difficulties which they have experienced and find it easier to relate to the client. On the other hand, the experience of another carer who has been faced with a similar situation may result in the opposite effect. The carer may not want to be reminded of a painful experience and may try to avoid discussing the matter with the client.

Compassion should be viewed as a response from the carer to the person being cared for, that they sympathise and want to understand the person's situation.

Conscience

Conscience is defined by Roach (1987) as 'the ability to distinguish between right and wrong'. In her writing about conscience, Roach has said that:

'*Conscience* is an intentional response, deliberate, meaningful and rational.
Conscience is the caring person attuned to the moral nature of things.
Conscience is the call of care and manifests itself as care.
Professional caring is reflected in a mature conscience' (Roach, 1987).

Carers and care workers need to be able to use conscience in a constructive, reflective way. They usually care for people who are vulnerable, and who are sometimes dependent on them. Therefore, they need a strong sense of conscience to ensure that they always act in the best interests of their clients.

Carers and care workers are in a very powerful position in relation to the people they care for. People who don't have a strong conscience, or who don't use their conscience in the best interests of others, can, and do, get into situations where the individuals they are supposed to be caring for are, in fact, harmed and abused.

Commitment

Commitment is a quality that is expressed by carers and care workers through the way in which they provide care for another person. Individuals who are dependent on receiving care need to feel that those who care for them have a certain 'stickability' and dedication to their work. Commitment is the determined effort to 'be there' for the individual needing care. It is a quality that is closely related to reliability and consistency.

People who take on a care role need to commit themselves to managing their time and workload in the interests of the people they care for, and must continue to care when they are faced with difficult situations. This sort of quality cannot be learnt from a textbook.

Confidence

Confidence is a personal quality that carers and care workers need to possess themselves and need to bring out in the individuals they care for. Confident carers and care workers are self-assured without being arrogant, and can use their own confidence to establish trusting relationships with others.

Genuineness is important in inspiring confidence in others. To build confidence in the people they care for, carers and care workers need to show them that they are able to:

- show interest in them as people, i.e. listen to them and talk to them giving respect
- assess their needs with the appropriate care requirements
- help them in different and difficult situations
- carry out caring tasks within the appropriate time span
- practise confidentiality with regard to the intimate details of clients
- speak the truth to the client with compassion and sensitivity.

Competence

Competence has been defined as 'the demonstration of knowledge, skills and attitudes, required to perform a given task or act' (Walklin, 1991).

Carers and care workers should have appropriate knowledge and effective practical skills to carry out the caring tasks that they attempt. A competent carer should be able to demonstrate that they can:

- provide a safe, clean, user-friendly environment for clients and service users
- assess the individual physical, intellectual, cognitive, emotional, social, cultural and religious needs of a client and act accordingly
- communicate with sensitivity, knowing when to speak and when to listen
- carry out the necessary practical tasks, such as washing, handling, toileting and feeding, in such a way that the client's dignity is maintained

ACTIVITY

Now that you know about the five Cs in caring and have thought about qualities for caring:

a) Review your own ideas and those of Roach (1987) and try to define what you believe are the essential qualities needed for caring.

b) Reflect on, and discuss, the extent to which you possess and need to develop your own caring qualities.

- promote a client's autonomy and independence and encourage them to make decisions.

Work experience and training can help carers and care workers to develop competence. In addition to this, it allows them to learn about the theories involved in caring. This helps them to see the relevance of the tasks that they carry out. Furthermore, competence is something that all carers and care workers should always be working towards. New and inexperienced carers and care workers should seek help and support to gradually build up their competence and should not undertake jobs or tasks that they are not competent to do.

EMPATHY

Empathy is an important skill to develop. A person who can empathise with another can understand their feelings and the situation they are in. However, it is important to say that empathy is more than just a 'fellow feeling'. It is the ability to see the situation from the other person's point of view. This may or may not be the result of one's own personal experience, personal contact with people, or student research into a particular subject. While it is true to say that a person who has suffered a bereavement is in the best position to empathise with another in a similar situation, a carer can support this person by trying to put themselves in a similar position and thinking what it means to that person and how they might feel if it happened to them.

However, if a carer has not experienced the situation or difficulty, it is important that they are honest about this and show that they are trying to understand and show care for the person. This aspect of empathy needs to be clarified, as in some situations a well-meaning person may say 'I understand just how you feel' when they have not been in the same position. This can cause negative, i.e. frustrated and angry, reactions in the person they are trying to help. Reinforcing the care and support by saying, for example, 'I have not been in your position, but I am here for you' is a more effective way of showing empathy. This also eliminates the possibility of a carer having to be 'all things to all people', which can be very stressful when they have several clients in their care.

Carers and care workers who work with a wide variety of people with a range of different situations, experiences and problems, will see that people have different responses to, and ways of coping with, situations. As it is unlikely that a carer or care worker will have had the same experiences as all their clients, it is useful to have some strategies to hand for developing empathy. They can:

- take time to listen to the client and allow them to talk about their situation – sometimes people find it easier to talk to someone outside their immediate family

- respond to the client, verbally and non-verbally, to show that they are listening and appreciate what is being said and experienced – a reassuring touch of the hand can make a difference

- try to appreciate what it must be like to be in the cared-for person's position
- show compassion and sympathise with the client during a difficult time
- be aware of the client's needs and help to fulfil them
- be aware of the client's non-verbal communication – it may tell you something that isn't being said
- put the client in touch with support or self-help groups, if the client is willing – these groups in turn can put the client in touch with someone who has a similar experience and who can help to support them.

CASE STUDY
Alice

Alice, aged 87, has just been admitted to a residential nursing home. A few hours after admission, she is telling the care assistants, 'I shouldn't be here, you know. I'm not going to get home now, am I? I feel terrible.'

1 What might you say to demonstrate your empathy for Alice at this moment?

2 How would you help Alice to settle into her new surroundings?

SELF-AWARENESS

Caring qualities can be developed through **self-awareness** – an important quality needed for care work. It involves:

- being aware of your own strengths and weaknesses as a person
- having the ability to identify and cope with your own feelings in circumstances that are sometimes difficult or upsetting
- being aware of your own attitudes and values and the ways in which these can affect others
- having the ability to keep your personal life separate from your role as a carer.

Self-awareness enables carers to develop their care practice. Carers often find it easier to highlight their weaknesses and under-estimate their strengths. Through exploring their strengths and weaknessess, carers can learn to build on their strengths to develop different areas of their care practice

Self-awareness is important because it enables a care worker to:

- *build up their confidence* through reviewing strengths and weaknesses. Learning to build on strengths and finding strategies to develop weaker areas can enhance a carer's self-esteem and the view that they have of themselves as a care worker
- *be in touch with their feelings* and therefore be more effective in how they relate to others within care relationships

ACTIVITIES

1 Ask yourself the question 'Do I like people?' Discuss why this is important in caring for others.

2 a) Make a list of your own strengths and weaknesses in relation to caring for others.

b) Discuss your list with a partner, concentrating on ways in which you can build on your strengths and develop your weaknesses to become an effective carer.

- *develop a more sensitive and flexible approach* to their work, allowing them to review their practice, have a realistic understanding of their competence, and focus on the ways in which they work with clients and colleagues.

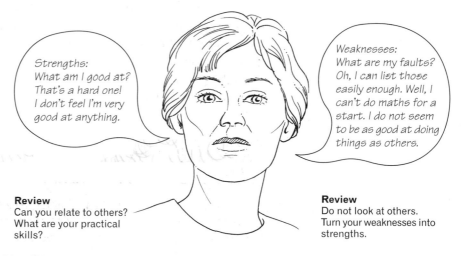

Identifying strengths and weaknesses

KEY POINT

Self-awareness is a key quality needed for development by any carer. Philip Burnard, a researcher and trainer in counselling and self-awareness, defines it as 'the process of getting to know your feelings, attitudes and values. It is also about the effect that you have on others' (Burnard, 1992).

A carer should always try to be aware of how they affect the people they work with. For example, clients can be particularly sensitive to a carer's moods. Clients can easily feel excluded, insecure and unhappy when a care worker expresses their own negative feelings or mood, even though it is unrelated to what they think or feel about the client. This does not mean that care workers should always appear cheerful. They should simply be aware that they need to manage and express their own feelings carefully. In circumstances where a client is in severe pain and distress, an over-cheerful care worker can be seen as very insensitive.

Self-awareness does not mean that a carer is constantly looking inwards after every word and action. It is a quality that should enable a carer to constructively review and reflect on their care practice and their relationship and interaction with clients and colleagues.

COMMUNICATION SKILLS

Communication is the ability to discuss, listen and exchange information with others. Effective communication is an essential requirement in caring and a vital skill that all carers and care workers need to develop.

Carers and care workers need to be able to:

- *listen* to others, to what they say and how they say it
- *ask questions and hold conversations* with a variety of people in different care situations
- *use a variety of forms of communication,* such as report writing, using the Internet and e-mail, as well as the telephone.

To communicate effectively, it is important to be aware of **non-verbal communication** – body language (gestures and postures), facial expression, use of personal space, body contact. Communication is a two-way process, i.e. for it to be effective the participants need to be able to listen and respond appropriately.

Listening skills

Learning to listen, making positive gestures towards the person speaking or making sympathetic sounds at appropriate points in the listening process are viewed as essential caring skills. Individuals who use care services usually expect that their carers should have the skills to listen in most situations. In order to listen effectively it is good practice to:

- sit or stand in a position that enables the individual to see and feel that they are being listened to, keep an 'open position', i.e. not folding your arms or crossing your legs
- make and maintain eye contact that demonstrates to the client that they are being listened to
- control facial expressions so that whatever is being said can be seen as important
- be patient and give the individual time to express what they want to say. This is particularly important when the person has a speech impairment, or if English is not their first language.

Listening skills are an important part of the assessment process in care settings. Assessment involves identifying the individual needs of the client. It can include questioning family and friends, listening and recording their responses so that the client's needs are identified.

Listening is also a valuable tool through which a carer can give positive reinforcement to those for whom they care. Clients and patients feel better when they believe that someone has listened to what they have said, their problems, their needs and their news.

> **ACTIVITY**
>
> In pairs, carry out this listening skills exercise:
>
> a) Partner 1 should talk about a topic for 2 minutes.
> b) Partner 2 will listen to what is being said. Written notes should not be taken, but partner 2 should concentrate on what is being said. Afterwards partner 2 will share an account of the topic with a larger group.
>
> Change roles and carry out the task again.

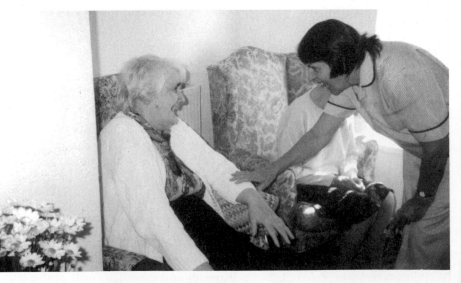

The carer conveys warmth as she listens to the client

According to Philip Burnard (1992) listening has three aspects that skilled care workers and carers should develop and learn to apply in their own practice:

- *linguistic aspects*, which involve listening to the words, phrases and metaphors and taking a general note of what is being said
- *paralinguistic aspects*, which involve being aware of the timing, volume, pitch, accent, fluency of what is being said. The care worker should listen with more depth to what is being said and how it is being said. This will involve the carer beginning to explore the perceptual world of the client and to build some empathy as they view the world from the client's perspective
- *non-verbal aspects*, which involve facial expression, use of gesture, touch, body position proximity, body movement and eye contact. At this level the carer is absorbing every detail of what is being said and making interpretations. The carer in this situation is beginning to mirror the feelings of the client.

Verbal communication skills

Talking to clients and asking appropriate questions is a key skill needed to identify a client's concerns and to find out how they are feeling. Carers should be sensitive to the way that they approach a client when gathering personal information.

The way in which a carer conducts a conversation and talks to a client is essential to the successful development of the relationship between them. Starting and maintaining conversations is not an easy thing for some people to do.

Talking does not just depend on the words being said. There are other considerations to be taken into account. These include:

- the tone of the voice
- the volume and pitch of the voice
- using hands and arms to express what is being said
- facial expressions and gestures
- eye contact.

Those new to caring may feel anxious at the thought of starting and maintaining a conversation and they may feel that they lack the necessary confidence. In order to develop verbal communication skills, especially to do with managing conversations:

- try to introduce yourself with warmth and a smile
- always welcome people using their name. If in doubt, ask the person their name
- make it a rule to try to remember names – use a pocket notebook if this proves to be a problem. Check these notes to reinforce your memory before meeting a client or colleague
- ask a simple introductory question to get a conversation started. For example:

– How are you today?

– Are you warm enough?

– Is there anything that I can do for you?

- if maintaining conversation is difficult, use positive gestures and facial expressions.

Carers can develop their expertise in using conversation and other verbal skills by talking and listening to clients, by monitoring the reactions of others in different situations and by evaluating their own practice. However, it is important to realise that the behaviour of others can have an effect through no fault of the carer.

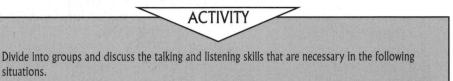

ACTIVITY

Divide into groups and discuss the talking and listening skills that are necessary in the following situations.

- You work in a nursery and have been asked to set up a session with a group of four children aged 3 years, to talk about their pets or the pets they would like to have. How would you set up the session and what would you do?

- You work in a day centre for older people. A group of them are sitting together, but not talking. They are Maud, who is 75, Sid aged 80, Fred aged 69, Jean aged 70 and Beth who is 73. How would you start the conversation, what would you say and how would you say it? What strategies might you need to use to keep the conversation going?

Barriers to communication

It is important to look at behaviour which can hinder effective communication between individuals. Barriers to communication can be caused by:

- carers and clients having fixed and stereotypical attitudes and behaviour, reinforced by negative gestures and body language

- one person dominating the conversation and not giving time for others to speak

- outbursts of impatience, screaming, tears and anger

- the feelings of one person being projected onto another because that person reminds them of somebody they know. This can either be someone they liked or someone they disliked or who caused them pain. These circumstances can have either a positive or negative effect on the communication process. This is called 'transference' – a term used by the psychologist Sigmund Freud. It is important to recognise that transference can occur – a carer may find they instantly dislike a client or service user as it reminds them of someone they know, or vice versa

- feelings of inadequacy or fear of failure on the part of the carer, which limit the way in which they can relate to their clients

- carers who are overwhelmed by their own problems, and so find it hard to deal with the problems of others

- a memory or feeling that may suddenly be remembered triggering a reaction such as a feeling of instability and frustration
- a carer refusing to react in a situation with a client because they cannot believe that there is anything to worry about – known as a 'blind spot'
- apathy and boredom which is expressed through non-verbal communication.

CASE STUDY

Bill

In a busy outpatients' department of a cancer hospital an older patient recognises a ward nurse who cared for him during a recent stay in hospital. He calls out to her as she walks through outpatients. She says 'Hello Bill, how are you?' He replies 'I've had a bad morning. I got up early and I was very sick. I don't know how long my wife can cope, and my daughter lives so far away. Then as I was shaving I passed blood and I don't know what to do'. The nurse replies 'Oh never mind, you'll get over it.'

1 How do you think Bill might feel after this conversation?

2 How do you think the nurse feels?

3 What are the key issues that affect the conversation?

4 Are there any barriers in communication in this case study? If so, what are they?

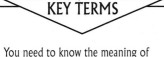

KEY TERMS

You need to know the meaning of the following words and phrases. Go back through the chapter to make sure that you understand them.

barriers to communication
empathy
five Cs of caring
non-verbal communication
self-awareness

In summary, by developing the qualities and skills which are necessary to support the caring process, carers and care workers can reinforce existing skills and learn new skills.

Values for caring

This chapter addresses the significance of values in caring and the importance attached to challenging prejudices and discriminatory behaviour in the way that caring is practised. The key topics covered in this chapter are:

- Values and principles in caring
- Support through effective communication
- Confidentiality and privacy
- Respect for rights and personal choices
- Respect for personal beliefs
- Anti-discriminatory care.

People who are involved in caring for individuals, formally or informally, usually have some idea about what good care is. Sometimes these ideas are vague and blurred and people simply try to do their best for the individuals they are caring for. Despite beginning with good intentions, it is possible for carers to lose sight of what they are trying to achieve and to become involved in providing mediocre and even poor standards of care. People get into these situations when they lack knowledge and understanding of important care values and when they fail to apply these values in their practice.It is therefore necessary to review the values and principles which underpin care practice.

VALUES AND PRINCIPLES IN CARING

A value is a belief about what is morally right and important. *The Oxford Dictionary of Current English* (1985) defines values as 'principles or standards, one's judgement of what is important in life'.

People involved in caring for others are expected to hold a number of important values and to apply these when they carry out care. Adams (1994) says that when values are applied in caring they are used as principles to guide day-to-day care practice. These key values are known as the **Care Value Base**.

The Care Value Base is expressed in terms of client rights. Where it is properly applied, the value base ensures that people who need care are treated equally and fairly in terms of their individual rights. These include the right to:

- support through effective communication
- **confidentiality** and **privacy**
- have individual's choices respected
- have personal beliefs acknowledged and acted upon
- receive **anti-discriminatory care**.

Each of these values, and the ways in which they are applied as principles, are discussed in this chapter. There are a number of opportunities to reflect on what is being said. Activities are provided to encourage and develop a clearer understanding of the values and principles involved.

Understanding the different elements within the Care Value Base forms a strong foundation for carers and care workers to more fully appreciate the rights of clients. First, however, it is important to recognise the reasoning behind the need to establish values and principles in care practice. We need to start by reviewing the meaning of attitudes and behaviour.

Attitudes and behaviour

Attitudes are the result of the ways in which individuals form opinions. They can reflect the positive or negative thinking of an individual. A person's attitudes affect the way they behave in given situations.

Exploring the way in which attitudes can affect behaviour can be a useful exercise for carers and care workers. When faced with situations in which they do not agree with the client with regard to their beliefs or lifestyle, carers and care workers must learn that the client has rights which should be supported as part of their care practice.

When attitudes to different issues and individuals become fixed and inflexible, this can lead to stereotyping.

Stereotyping

A **stereotype** is a fixed view a person has about another person or group of people. The person has a fixed set of attitudes which are linked to certain (often inaccurate) characteristics of individuals or groups of people. For example, older people may be grouped together and viewed as a 'drain of society' because of the increasing cost of their care. The disconcerting aspect of stereotypical attitudes is that they can often affect the way in which a person thinks about others. Sometimes these attitudes can influence the way in which a person relates to issues outside their personal experience.

Stereotyping can lead to:

- **labelling** – the way in which a person or group is believed to display a set of characteristics which are based on the (often inaccurate) assumptions and attitudes of others
- **prejudice** – often defined as 'prejudgement which relates closely to fixed attitudes and which can result in **discrimination** and disempowerment', i.e. issues which relate to lack of choice, opportunity and personal rights (Moonie *et al.*, 1995).

Prejudice and discrimination are discussed further under *Anti-discriminatory care*, page 30.

A question which is frequently asked is 'How are stereotypes formed?' There are various theories, based on two distinct ideas, which suggest that they may arise from:

- early **socialisation** and learning experiences, personality traits and the general psychological processes involved in attitude formation
- prejudiced attitudes and adverse labelling by others which may result in low self-esteem and a self-fulfilling prophecy of low achievement.

It can be seen, therefore, that both prejudice and labelling have a negative effect on how people relate to themselves and to others.

Exploring how attitudes can affect the way in which one person behaves to another is an important part of self-awareness, discussed in Chapter 2 (page 16). Within the caring process, fixed attitudes, prejudice and labelling of others may lead a carer giving one client less attention than another. Therefore, an understanding of the different elements of the Care Value Base forms a strong foundation for carers and care workers to appreciate more fully the rights of clients.

SUPPORT THROUGH EFFECTIVE COMMUNICATION

Effective communication is a key feature of the care relationship. A carer who is an effective communicator is somebody who can build supportive relationships with the individuals they are caring for.

There are many different ways in which effective care relationships can be developed through good communication. These include the following.

- Introduce yourself to the individuals you are caring for. Find out early on in the relationship the name by which they want to be addressed. Not everyone wishes to be called by their first name.
- Talk to clients at *their* level of understanding and avoid being patronising or talking down to them.
- Convey warmth, interest and take time to listen to what the client is saying. Try not to start a conversation if you do not have time to stop and chat.
- Show empathy if you have any experience of what the client is facing, but always show concern in a non-patronising way.

- Encourage a client to talk about their wishes and needs.
- Greet clients at the beginning of a shift and say goodbye at the end of a shift.

Care workers and carers can support clients by providing them with relevant information and by promoting their right to be involved in their own care and in the relevant decision-making process. However, there are difficulties which may arise relating to **challenging behaviour** – demanding or threatening behaviour, outbursts of verbal abuse and stubbornness which can be accompanied by aggressive and violent actions.

Coping with challenging behaviour

When clients have suffered a number of changes in their lives, and also may suffer from a debilitating disorder, they may be affected by bouts of anger and frustration. They can feel desperately anxious about their future, long for the past or feel depressed and hopeless. They may express this in challenging behaviour.

The safety of the clients themselves, as well as other clients and carers, has to be considered when managing challenging behaviour. There are a number of ways in which carers can cope with challenging behaviour.

- First, try to defuse the situation, talk calmly, being aware of any dangers to other people.
- Never lose your temper or raise your voice to shout loudly at the person you are caring for.
- Discuss the situation with other members of the team.
- Don't be afraid to ask for help. Seek advice if and when necessary.
- Reflect on the incidents of challenging behaviour and try to identify any triggers in your own, or other people's, verbal comments or body language that may have led to the negative behaviour in the first place.
- Write up a factual report of the incident.

CASE STUDY

Jake

Jake is a 17-year-old student who is spending his first placement at a residential home for older people. He has no previous experience of working with older people. When he tries to serve lunch to Maisie, an 83-year-old resident, she refuses to take it and throws it on the floor. Later she shouts at his supervisor that Jake did not give her any lunch, and that he threw it on the floor. Her main carer is off duty. Jake feels upset and tries to explain what happened to the supervisor.

1   What is happening in this situation? Why might Maisie be refusing food from Jake?

2   How should the supervisor react in this situation?

3   Suggest some strategies for Jake.

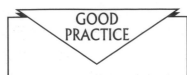

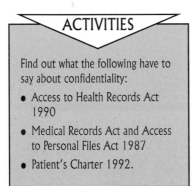

ACTIVITIES

Find out what the following have to say about confidentiality:

- Access to Health Records Act 1990
- Medical Records Act and Access to Personal Files Act 1987
- Patient's Charter 1992.

CONFIDENTIALITY AND PRIVACY

Maintaining confidentiality and privacy are key principles in care practice. It is an important requirement for carers and care workers to understand the different issues which relate to confidentiality and privacy.

Confidentiality

Confidentiality is not about keeping secrets. It is an underlying principle of health and social care practice which ensures that information about an individual's health and personal life is respected and protected.

Miller (1996) says 'it is about the appropriateness of sharing, transmitting and storing information about a service user when a number of competing factors may influence decisions about information use'.

The Access to Health Records Act (1990) sets out the law governing an individual's rights to see files and records that contain written information about them. There are some circumstances in which a person may be denied access to some parts of their records. According to the document *Working Together under the Children Act* (1989), in some areas of child protection, any decision 'to withhold or disclose information should be able to be justified. Practitioners should always take the opportunity to discuss the matter fully with other practitioners, and explore the ramifications or the outcomes of their decisions'.

Clarke, Sachs and Ford (1995) explain that:

'care workers are never fully at liberty to keep secrets between themselves and clients, as the worker is representing his or her organisation and may need to inform specific individuals of any critical information, particularly where clients and others may be at risk.'

Care workers should always explain their organisation's confidentiality procedure, and its limits, to the person they are caring for.

Carers and care workers should be particularly careful about breaching confidentiality when they talk about their work. Informal chats in coffee breaks, on public transport travelling to and from work or any indiscreet conversations with family and friends should be avoided. All of these can be passed on to others and eventually may be passed back to the client.

The principle of confidentiality frequently raises dilemmas when the health and safety of others, as well as that of the person receiving care, is involved. Despite this, maintaining a person's privacy and confidentiality is an essential requirement in terms of building and reinforcing professional relationships between clients and their carers.

Carers and care workers are in a privileged position – they have access to information about other people that is often very personal and sensitive. It is a betrayal of trust to disclose this information to others who are not directly involved in the person's care, unless the individual gives you permission to do so. Confidentiality influences the way in which relationships between carers and the individuals they care for develop and grow. When a person discloses information that is confidential, they trust the person they are telling not to make this public outside of the care team. Relationships cannot develop without this trust.

CASE STUDY

Martin and Jane

Martin and Jane are in their late twenties and have recently moved to London from a city in the north of England. They have a 6-year-old son, Simon, and 2-year-old daughter, Amy. Martin and Jane were once both dependent on heroin, which they injected using a shared needle. They recently found out that they are both HIV positive. The family has now settled in London and needs to register with a GP. Simon will require a local school.

Research and discuss your answers to the following questions:

1 Is it necessary for Martin and Jane to declare their health status, i.e. being HIV positive, to a new health authority?

2 Who are the health and social care professionals who would be involved in this case?

3 Should Simon's school be involved? If so, why?

4 What about Amy? If she is registered at a nursery, should her parents' health status be declared?

5 What are the issues of confidentiality once this family registers with a GP?

6 Find out about the different types of care in your area available for people who are HIV positive. Does your local authority have a special unit which offers support, counselling and confidential advice?

Privacy

Privacy is defined as the right of an individual to their own personal space. The environment of care settings, such as residential and nursing homes and hospitals, can be impersonal and can restrict opportunities for privacy. This is particularly the case where individuals do not have separate bedrooms, where they share bathroom facilities or use communal lounge and dining areas. It is important that people who provide care services make every effort to promote and maintain privacy, even in difficult circumstances.

Carers and care workers should never presume that they have automatic access to an individual's room. They should always knock and wait for a reply before entering. Even where a person has to be helped to use the toilet or bath, it is important that a carer or care worker avoids invading the person's privacy by walking in and out of the bathroom without getting the individual's permission. Invading privacy breaches an important principle of care practice.

RESPECT FOR RIGHTS AND PERSONAL CHOICES

Rights

Respect for the worth and dignity of every individual is a key value in caring (Miller, 1996). Carers and care workers should acknowledge and express this value in the ways that they provide care. People who use care services, or who are in receipt of informal care, share the same human and legal rights and protection as other people in society.

Those who depend on care services should never experience abuse, exploitation or neglect from the person, or people, caring for them. They should always have their rights, choices and views acknowledged, encouraged and supported. These should be an integral part of the quality of care, regardless of a person's race, social class, background, sexuality, beliefs, gender, cognitive, mental or physical ability.

Choices

It is often the responsibility of the carer to identify and agree with the client their preferred choices in terms of the care, treatment and support that they require.

Choices can be about 'big' issues such as whether, or when, to go into hospital or receive treatment, or about 'smaller', but no less important matters, such as the food or clothing that a person would prefer on a particular day.

Promoting choice

Promoting choice gives a person real options – they are able to make an independent decision about which option they prefer. Part of caring is about promoting an individual's right to have choices and supporting their decisions when they exercise their right and make those choices. People who are able to make decisions for themselves are said to have **autonomy**.

Preventing choice

In some situations, however, carers and care workers may reduce or prevent a client's choices. One of the consequences of giving choices to individuals who receive care is that they sometimes choose options that carers and care workers do not agree with or which they believe are risky. Carers need to ensure that they do not over-protect clients, and thereby reduce their autonomy. The idea that the carer and the care worker know what is best for the client is known as paternalism. People should not be prevented from participating in activities in care settings by paternalistic staff. All people should be able to make choices that involve reasonable and responsible risk-taking.

Carers and care workers should continually review the strategies of care they use with each client with regard to the degree of **empowerment** they have, i.e. the amount of control they have over their own life, their rights and choices. When someone is not capable of making choices because they have a cognitive or mental disability, this should not reduce the choices or rights of that individual. In some cases an **advocate** can be assigned to a person to represent their interests and to speak on their behalf, if they cannot speak for themselves.

CASE STUDY

Sanjit

Sanjit is a 45-year-old Pakistani man who has suffered a stroke. He is in the early stages of rehabilitation. He now attends physiotherapy to restore movement to the muscles on the left side of his body. He feels very depressed as he was a successful business man before the stroke and now feels that his life has become very empty. He is due to be discharged home from hospital. His wife is very concerned about him.

As a care worker:

1 What strategies would you use to help Sanjit come to terms with his situation?

2 What would you do to encourage Sanjit to make decisions about his future?

3 How would you develop his autonomy?

RESPECT FOR PERSONAL BELIEFS

Accepting people without judging them or making assumptions about them is a key principle in caring. People who are employed as care workers are expected to accept unconditionally the individuals they care for. This does not mean that a care worker has to accept or condone hostile, aggressive or other anti-social behaviour or attitudes from those in their care. It does mean that, whilst a carer can reject a person's behaviour as being unacceptable, they should never reject the person themselves or deny their need for help.

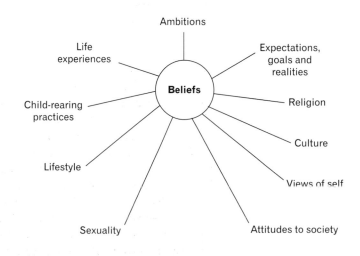

Factors which form an individual's belief system

Acknowledging a person's beliefs is a key part of accepting them as a person. Beliefs:

- relate closely to an individual's perception of who they are – their identity
- underpin their attitudes, views, religious affiliation, cultural needs, political persuasion, their moral and ethical views, as well as their sexual orientation.

Showing respect for an individual's beliefs really amounts to showing respect for the person themself. This has an impact on the individual's level of self-esteem.

A person will often reveal the nature of their beliefs through what they say in conversation and through the ways that they behave. An individual's belief system will influence their thoughts and ideas about a range of matters including:

- their expectations of, and goals in, life
- attitudes to society
- religion
- sexuality
- cultural identity and needs
- lifestyle
- views of self
- child-rearing practices.

It is not unusual for carers and care workers to find that their belief systems are different to those they are caring for. In these situations the person providing care should always:

- respect the other person's views and give them the opportunity to discuss issues when necessary
- show support and care through listening skills, body language and by making constructive comments
- recognise that the person's beliefs are central to their view of themself and support them in expressing religious and cultural beliefs that are important to them.

▼ ACTIVITY ▼

In small groups, discuss and make a list of different factors and experiences that can influence the development of a person's beliefs.

ANTI-DISCRIMINATORY CARE

All people involved in caring for others should practise **anti-discriminatory care**. This is a key principle in good care practice. Anti-discriminatory care practice involves being:

- aware of different forms of unfair discrimination
- sensitive to the individual's ethnic background and cultural needs
- prepared actively to challenge and work towards reducing the unfair discrimination experienced by clients and carers within a care setting.

The basis of discrimination

Prejudice and ignorance, i.e. views formed with a lack of knowledge and awareness, tend to underpin discriminatory behaviour (see page 24).

A prejudice is a negative, hostile, stereotypical belief about a group of people that is applied to an individual who belongs to, or appears to be a member of, that group. For example, some people hold prejudices about what 'women's work' should and should not involve, about the skills and abilities of black people or about the personal qualities of individuals with a homosexual orientation.

Forms of discrimination

A person who is discriminated against experiences unfair treatment because of prejudice, intolerance and ignorance. People tend to discriminate against others who are, or seem to be, different from them in some way. People from many different situations, cultures and backgrounds can be subject to discrimination.

There are different forms of discrimination:

- *direct discrimination (overt discrimination)* – occurs when intentional and obvious unfair treatment or behaviour is directed towards another person or group of people. An example might be racist jokes being directed at a particular individual

- *indirect discrimination (covert discrimination)* – occurs when the unfair treatment or behaviour towards another person or group of people is not obvious, and sometimes not even intended, but is evident in different ways. Low numbers of women, or people from ethnic minorities, or people with disabilities, in senior and management positions in care organisations can sometimes be an indication of indirect discrimination. It may be that the structure and procedures of the organisation make it harder for people from these groups to benefit from promotion opportunities.

Discrimination can take the form of unfair treatment because of race (racism), gender (sexism), age (ageism), disability, sexuality, religion, health status, cognitive ability or political persuasion.

Carers can exhibit discriminatory behaviour in a variety of ways. For example by:

- avoiding contact with a particular person. This can be difficult if the person is part of a team, or a client being cared for in a small residential unit

- ignoring the person, not looking in their direction, not having eye contact, not listening when they make conversation, generally being disinterested

- making remarks and comments which are disrespectful and spiteful

- highlighting a person's difficulties, weaknesses, drawing attention to these in conversation, making comments about a person's disability or social role.

Insensitive and discriminatory attitudes cause much anguish, particularly if the client is dependent and unable to move round and extend their contact with others. On the other hand, it can be just as difficult if a client takes an obvious dislike to a carer and makes remarks which are hurtful or indiscrete.

Challenging discrimination

Challenging discrimination is difficult in care settings, especially where the people who are doing the discriminating are colleagues. However, where a care worker identifies discriminatory practice, they should explore the reasoning behind this, or any incident that occurs, and challenge the person or people concerned. If discrimination remains unchallenged, it can reinforce prejudices and make them stronger, and so a vicious circle begins (see the diagram below).

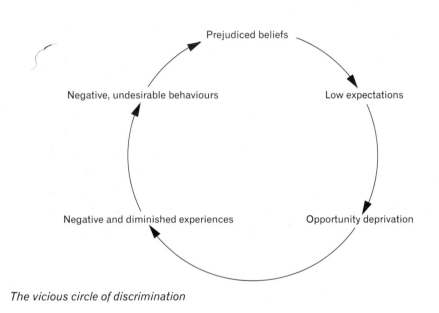

The vicious circle of discrimination

CASE STUDY

Janet

Janet is 80. She has experienced a stroke, is now confined to a wheelchair, and is in full-time residential care. She finds that when Chloe, one of the care workers, is on duty and assigned to her floor she has to wait longer than others for help with personal care, especially toileting. She feels that Chloe does not like her. This is happening several times a day. She does not like to complain as she fears the situation will get worse.

1 As a carer, how would you assess whether Chloe's behaviour is discriminatory?

2 What are the effects of this situation on Janet?

3 Would you challenge Chloe's behaviour?

ACTIVITIES

1 Carry out some research on the list of legislation. Find out how each one supports anti-discriminatory practice in health and social care settings. Present your findings in a table.

2 Research and read any relevant government reports that support anti-discriminatory practice in health and social care. Make notes of your findings.

Copies of legislation may be found in local libraries or are available from the Stationery Office. Textbooks may contain some information, as well as the Internet and CD-ROMs.

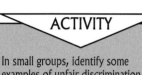

ACTIVITY

In small groups, identify some examples of unfair discrimination which take place in different care settings. Describe how these can affect the behaviour of clients towards carers or of carers towards clients. Remember that, if you are discussing real incidents, you should protect the confidentiality of your clients by not using their real names.

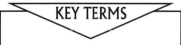

KEY TERMS

You need to know the meaning of the following words and phrases. Go back through the chapter and make sure you understand them.

advocate
anti-discriminatory care
autonomy
Care Value Base
challenging behaviour
confidentiality
discrimination
empowerment
labelling
prejudice
privacy
socialisation
stereotype

The vicious circle works on the assumption that everyone feels the same about different issues. This adds weight to the argument and leads to a continued circle of fixed attitudes and negative behaviour patterns. By identifying the effects of the vicious circle, it is possible to intervene and retrain or change attitudes.

Anti-discrimination legislation

Policies, procedures and legislation have been set up to protect the individual from unfair treatment in care situations. Legislation that supports anti-discriminatory practice includes:

- Chronically Sick and Disabled Persons Act 1970
- Equal Pay Act 1970
- Equal Pay Amendment Act 1983
- Sex Discrimination Act 1975, revised in 1986
- Race Relations Act 1976
- Children Act 1989
- Education (Handicapped Children) Act 1980
- Mental Health Act 1983
- Disabled Persons Act 1981 and 1986
- National Health Service and Community Care Act 1990
- Criminal Justice Act and Public Order Act 1994
- Disability Discrimination Act 1995
- Carers and Services Recognition Act 1995.

Equal opportunities legislation should be put into practice through the equal opportunity policies that care settings develop. These give care providers an ideal way of reviewing their anti-discriminatory care practice. Whatever the care setting, patients, clients or service users are entitled to equality of care, with their individual basic needs being met in a non-discriminatory way. Equal opportunities policies, charters and legislation aim to put this into practice.

It is important to understand that anti-discriminatory practice is not based on the idea of everybody being treated the same. It is more about recognising that everyone is an individual with different needs, and addressing these different and individual needs of clients. For example, acknowledging and valuing individual differences in race, class, gender, age, disability and health status is an integral part of caring.

Identifying and being aware of social and cultural differences in society is a way of meeting the variety of individual needs that include religious and cultural as well as physical, intellectual, social and emotional requirements.

Anti-discriminatory care aims to identify and challenge fixed stereotypical attitudes and prejudice. It highlights people's assumptions and labelling systems that can deny or deprive clients of the high quality of care to which they are entitled.

Holistic care

PREVIEW

This chapter introduces the concept of **holistic care** and describes what is involved in providing individualised holistic care in any care setting. The key topics covered in this chapter are:

- Needs
- Physical needs
- Emotional needs
- Social needs
- Intellectual and cognitive needs
- Cultural needs
- Spiritual needs.

Holistic care is an approach to the caring process which assesses and meets all the different needs of an individual. This means that the care being given recognises the requirements of the whole person – their physical, intellectual and cognitive, social, emotional, spiritual and cultural needs.

Often the medical profession, i.e. doctors and nurses, are criticised for treating a disease or disorder rather than the person who is suffering. Holistic care explores other areas, such as the hopes, fears and beliefs of individuals, and these are considered alongside their illness.

Holistic care, therefore, recognises that people differ. It requires carers and care workers to discover a person's fears and hopes in order to support their individual personal developmental needs.

NEEDS

Every living thing, human, animal and plant, has basic needs which must be met in order for them to survive. These needs include:

- *physical needs* – relating to the body and how it works
- *social needs* – meeting others, making friends
- *emotional needs* – feeling of acceptance and security
- *intellectual and cognitive needs* – learning and educational needs
- *cultural needs* – individual cultural expectations and realities
- *spiritual needs* – fulfilling a belief or realisation of self-fulfilment through one means or another.

Abraham Maslow (1970), a psychologist, described human needs in terms of a hierarchy (see the diagram below). He considered that humans have basic needs which must be met if the person is to survive. When these basic requirements have been met, the person can consider higher needs. For instance, the person who feels cold, hungry and tired will seek warmth, food and rest before self-fulfilment or status.

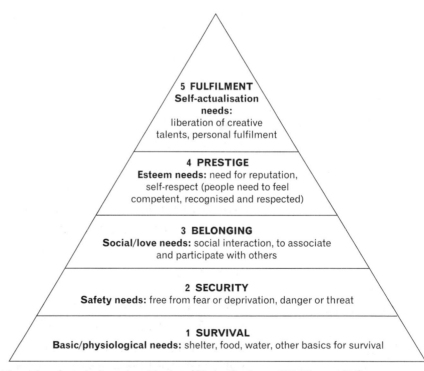

A hierarchy of needs, based on Maslow (Clarke, Sachs and Waltham, 1994)

Identifying needs

Before a carer and care worker can meet a client's needs, they must be able to identify them. It is important for care workers that they have a framework to assess an individual's needs. The most commonly used framework was

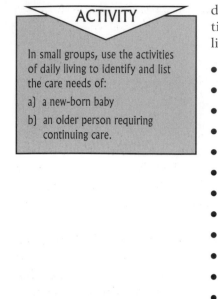

ACTIVITY

In small groups, use the activities of daily living to identify and list the care needs of:

a) a new-born baby

b) an older person requiring continuing care.

developed by Roper, Logan and Tierney in 1990 and is based on the activities carried out to support daily living. These are known as activities of daily living and are:

- maintaining a safe environment
- communication
- breathing
- eating and drinking
- eliminating
- personal cleansing and dressing
- controlling body temperature
- mobilising
- sleeping
- religious needs
- expressing sexuality
- wounds and dressings
- dying.

ACTIVITY

Investigate the strategies that Government and care agencies have implemented with regard to meeting the heating needs of older peole who live in their own homes.

PHYSICAL NEEDS

The physical needs of clients and service users cut across age groups, abilities or disabilities, race, gender and issues of social class. All individuals have the following physical needs which form part of their daily routines (care procedures). They need:

- to be warm and clothed
- to be healthy and to have a safe and secure place to live
- food to maintain a healthy diet
- rest, sleep and relaxation to promote good health
- to be able to wash and maintain their personal hygiene
- to be able to use a toilet
- to be able to exercise to keep the body supple and mobile as far as possible
- to have a stimulating environment in which to live and work.

Warmth and clothing

KEY POINT

Wearing appropriate clothes is very important to a client. If they are wearing comfortable, clean and well-fitting clothes, it can make them feel happier and more confident. It enhances their self-esteem and dignity.

Feeling warm is an essential requirement for all individuals. The body needs to maintain a certain temperature in order to survive. The heat-regulating system is stored in the part of the brain called the hypothalamus. When the body is cold, it shivers in order to generate heat to warm the body. When the body becomes warm and overheated, the blood rushes to the surface of the skin, which induces sweating. The body cools as the sweat evaporates on the skin surface. The normal body temperature ranges between 36–37 °C.

How different clients keep warm is explored in Part 2. However, clients living on their own, especially older people, may find keeping their homes warm a major financial concern, particularly in the winter months. Other vulnerable clients to which this applies are babies and young children, who

ACTIVITY

Choose one of the following clients and make a list of a suitable set of clothes, including underwear. Choose clothes suitable for either winter or summer. Give reasons why fabrics and styles were chosen. Describe how these clothes will be cared for.

- a baby age 6 months
- a child age 6 attending school
- a woman aged 34 who has multiple sclerosis
- a man aged 84 living in a residential home. He suffers from incontinence.

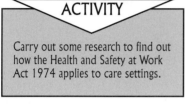

ACTIVITY

Carry out some research to find out how the Health and Safety at Work Act 1974 applies to care settings.

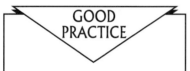

GOOD PRACTICE

There are precautions which carers can take as part of their role in providing a safe environment:

- A risk assessment should be carried out by a Health and Safety Officer to ensure the environment is safe.
- All equipment used should have regular safety checks.
- Cleaning agents, medicines, sharp and dangerous pieces of equipment should be locked away in secure storage.
- Lighting should be efficient and effective.
- Evacuation procedures in case of emergency or fire should be in place.
- Ventilation should be draught-free and should maintain a comfortable temperature.
- Furniture should be adjusted to match a client's abilities, for example, equipment for the

continued

can lose body heat very quickly in a cold environment. Therefore, it is not only important to monitor environmental warmth, but to ensure that clients are wearing adequate clothing.

Getting dressed is a focus to a client's day, whatever their age. A number of issues should be considered when choosing clothes with a client. Whenever possible, clients should always be involved in choosing what they should wear.

- *Fashion and style* Discuss with the client the different styles and materials available. If the client is in residential care, it is most convenient if their clothes are machine washable and crease-free. However, if the client has a particular favourite item of clothing which is linen, for example, specialised washing and ironing should be made available so that the client can wear it on special occasions.

- *Care of clothing* Caring for a client's clothes is important. Their clothing should be washed and ironed regularly. Clients in residential care should always be allowed to wear their own clothes, even if it means labelling each item. This is an integral part of their sense of identity and dignity.

- *Underwear* Items of underwear should be changed and washed regularly.

- *Protective clothing* Protective aprons/serviettes/bibs should be worn by clients at mealtimes if there is any prospect of them spilling food or if they are being fed.

- *Culture and dress* Clients from different cultures should be allowed to wear their own customary dress as it is an integral part of their cultural identity.

- *Adaptations and modifications of items of clothing* Clients with disabilities may need to have their clothes adapted. For example, clients with rheumatoid arthritis may need Velcro openings which are easier to manage than hooks and eyes or buttons.

- *Co-ordination of colour and style* Help clients to co-ordinate what they wear. Shoes should be included in this, and should be well fitted. Children's feet should be regularly measured by a professional shoe specialist.

- *Temperature variations* Clothes should be chosen bearing in mind the different seasons and variations in the weather.

Health and safety

The physical needs of an individual should raise issues of health and safety for both the carer and for those in their care. A service user needs to feel safe and all care providers should ensure that Health and Safety Regulations are adhered to. There are different health and safety regulations, including a risk assessment, which apply to different care settings (see Appendix 3).

Diet

Individuals need to eat and drink in order to survive. They need a healthy diet to maintain the growth and development of different parts of the body. A balanced **healthy diet** should provide sufficient energy (calories) to enable the person to maintain normal body weight. The diet should include daily amounts of fats, proteins, carbohydrates, vitamins, minerals, fibre, water, and trace elements.

visually impaired, chairs which give support to back and legs.
- Sufficient and suitable work surfaces should be clean, dust-free, easy to maintain and keep clean.
- A named qualified first aider and first aid box should be on-site and accessible in times of emergency (See Appendix 4).

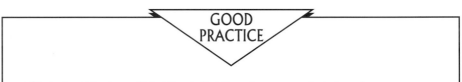

ACTIVITY

a) Research the function of each of the components of a healthy diet, and what happens if the diet is deficient in each one. Note which foods contain each component.
b) Find out what the recommended daily intake of each is (note that these vary with the age of the person).
c) Make a table of your findings using the following headings: Dietary component, Function, Deficiency disorder or disease, Source, Recommended daily intake.

The task of feeding clients can be time-consuming for a carer who has several clients to look after. Each carer should assess whether clients can effectively feed themselves and decide the degree of support which is necessary. There are some tasks common to all client groups which support good practice (see below).

Whenever possible, meal times should be very much a part of a client's routine and should be made to be as enjoyable as possible.

GOOD PRACTICE

- Clients should be given sufficient time to feed themselves, encouraging independence.
- Food should be prepared in a way that makes it easier for clients to feed themselves. If necessary it should be cut up and placed on a plate with a non-slip mat.
- The plate of food should be placed close to the client, within easy reach and with suitable cutlery.
- The food should be presented on the plate in an attractive way to promote the appetite. Do not allow the food to get cold.

Rest, sleep and relaxation

It is important to get enough rest and sleep in order to maintain a healthy body. During sleep, the body temperature falls and metabolism slows. The body produces hormones and growth factors, and repairs damage. People who are over-tired find it difficult to function well. Sick and vulnerable clients need more rest and sleep so that their bodies can heal and recover. Carers should integrate rest and sleep periods as part of the daily routine.

Carers and care workers can support an individual's healthy sleeping patterns. This will involve spending time finding out about a person's normal sleep pattern which will include:

- times for going to bed and getting up
- pre-bed time routine – the tasks and activities which a person performs before turning out the light. For instance, some people walk around their homes, locking up, filling a hot water bottle and making a hot drink before getting into bed, while others have a long soak in the bath, visit the toilet and get into bed with a book

- the number of hours a person feels they need to achieve a good night's sleep
- the number of hours a person sleeps and how they sleep. Are they restless? Do they wake up at regular intervals? Where a client is unable to speak for themselves, carers should ask relatives or a person who will speak on their behalf, i.e. an **advocate.**

Some people have difficulty sleeping at night, that is, they suffer from insomnia. There may be many reasons for this, such as stress, depression, having eaten a large meal before going to bed.

A carer should ensure that beds are comfortable and that the mattress is firm. Sufficient blankets should be provided and all noises kept to a minimum. Carers are also responsible for monitoring their clients as they sleep, checking that they are asleep, observing they are rested and relaxed.

Washing and personal hygiene

Washing is the part of a daily routine which involves the way in which an individual keeps themselves clean and maintains their personal hygiene. There are areas of the body which need special attention (see the diagram below).

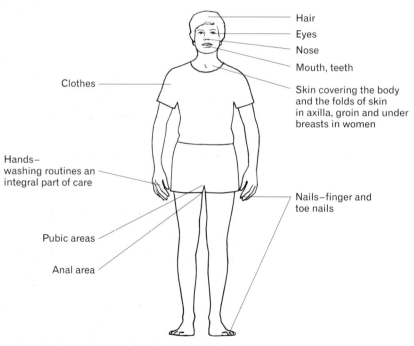

Areas for special attention when washing

Personal hygiene routines begin at birth and continue throughout the lifespan, involving:

- *washing, bathing and showering* – daily or every other day. These procedures ensure that the skin is washed clean of any dirt, debris and sweat. For individuals who are confined to bed, a blanket or bed bath will be carried out by the carer

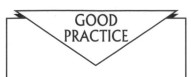

- *hair washing* – ensures that the individual's hair is kept clean, brushed and free from infestation, such as head lice or nits
- *nail care* – keeps nails short and clean. This includes both finger and toe nails
- *foot care* – washing feet and massaging feet encourages the blood supply. It keeps the skin supple and prevents soreness and infection between the toes.

How these routines are supported depends on factors such as:

- *family life and child-rearing practices* – the washing routines carried out by mothers or primary care givers
- *peer groups* – what is in fashion – a clean and glossy look or an unkempt and unwashed look
- *a person's financial status*, i.e. how much money they have to spend on soap, shampoo, heating water for a bath
- *social isolation*, for example, if they live on their own, an individual may not think that it is necessary to wash every day
- *culture* – different cultures have special requirements with regard to personal hygiene. For example, Muslims have ritual washing ceremonies several times a day. In addition, they use the right hand for clean tasks and the left for unclean tasks
- *ability to wash* – some disabilities, such as arthritis, can make washing difficult. With other disorders, such as depression, the client may not want to be bothered with washing.

CASE STUDY

Nicola

Nicola is a Health and Social Care student who is on work experience at a residential home for older people. One morning she arrives to find Dot in Room 12, sitting in a chair with wet underclothes. She tells Nicola that she has been ringing for a care assistant for hours. She has not had a wash. She could not wait for the toilet. She has the evidence of boiled egg on her jumper and crumbs round her mouth.

Discuss and decide the following:

1 What has happened in the case of Dot?

2 Prioritise Nicola's actions.

3 What routines should be in place with regard to personal hygiene?

Regular personal hygiene routines help to control the spread of infection. Good hand washing techniques are essential when carers work with more than one client. Carers should always wash their hands before and after working with individual clients. They should actively encourage clients to wash their hands before meals and after going to the toilet.

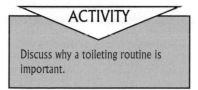

ACTIVITY

Discuss why a toileting routine is important.

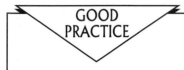

GOOD PRACTICE

Carers should ensure that toileting routines are set up in all care settings. These should include:
- correct labelling of client's nappies, underclothes and personal clothing
- equipment being available for hygiene procedures which are carried out with all clients, i.e. disposable gloves and handwashing facilities for the carer, disposable wipes and tissues, toileting area (toilets/potties, bedpan) and facilities for sterilisation
- privacy, i.e. cubicles with toilets, or a sectioned off area for potties. Doors should be capable of being shut, with or without safety locks, depending on the care setting
- procedures for waste disposal, i.e. for dirty nappies, used bedpans and urinals.

KEY POINT

Using exercise to increase or maintain mobility is an asset to any client. Those who have become immobile as a result of disease, disorder or dysfunction will view any ability to move and complete a physical task as an achievement.

There are certain other hygiene requirements which also apply to carers. These involve:

- maintaining personal hygiene requirements as for a client
- keeping jewellery to a minimum
- keeping nails short and clean
- wearing sensible and comfortable clothes if a uniform is not provided. Choose clothes which will accommodate the bending and stretching movements involved
- wearing shoes which are comfortable and practical, with low heels and without steel tips.

Supporting the personal hygiene routine is also an effective way of enabling a client to feel better. It retains their dignity and therefore maintains their sense of health and well-being. Individual client routines will be discussed in Chapters 6–10.

Toileting and elimination needs

Toileting is the method used to dispose of the body's waste products. The biological processes of human beings involve the elimination (or disposal) of waste products. The waste products are:

- urine, which is produced by the kidneys. The urine filters from the kidneys to the bladder. When the bladder is almost full, the bladder sends a message to the brain warning the person of the need to pass urine
- faeces, which are produced by the bowel. The faeces are the left-over products of digestion and, as with the bladder, when the bowel is nearly full, it sends a message to the brain warning the person of the need to empty the bowel.

Toileting begins at birth, with the primary care-giver carrying out the task of nappy changing. It continues with the potty training of a toddler, which encourages the young child to become independent. It is also an important part of learning the skills which are considered by society to be socially acceptable. However, there are clients who need regular support with toileting routines.

Toileting is a basic need. Training routines to ensure that a client can successfully carry out this task is an integral part of the caring process. More detail may be found in Chapters 6–10.

Exercise and mobility

Exercise is a method of promoting muscle and joint movement, encouraging the body to move and work in a co-ordinated way.

As a baby grows she strengthens her body and limbs and makes efforts to move, crawl, stand, walk and eventually run. This develops the gross motor skills of the body (large muscle movements) as well as the fine motor skills (manipulative muscle movements). As children grow into adults, their bodies grow and develop. Exercise continues to be necessary throughout the lifespan.

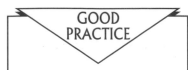

GOOD
PRACTICE

Exercises which promote mobility
are often devised by a
physiotherapist who will outline a
number of exercises for a client, or
group of clients, which can be
practised every day. The carer will
often be part of this programme and
should ensure that:

- sufficient time is given to the
  client to complete the exercises
  at their own pace
- help is given to the client using
  suitable aids, for example, a soft
  ball to place on the palm of the
  client's hand for them to
  squeeze, thus using and
  retraining the fine muscles in the
  hand
- assistance is available should the
  client feel that it is necessary
- praise and encouragement is
  given with each exercise that is
  carried out.

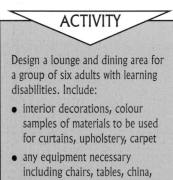

ACTIVITY

Design a lounge and dining area for
a group of six adults with learning
disabilities. Include:

- interior decorations, colour
  samples of materials to be used
  for curtains, upholstery, carpet
- any equipment necessary
  including chairs, tables, china,
  cutlery
- pictures, posters and mirrors.

CASE STUDY

Joe

Joe is 80. He has suffered a stroke and is paralysed down his left side. He
is discharged into a residential home for older people. You are his key
worker and main carer and it is your responsibility to encourage him to
exercise daily.

1 How would you go about planning the exercise sessions?

2 Describe the exercise programme that would be set up for Joe.

3 What equipment would be necessary to aid mobility?

The carer's role in promoting mobility is important simply because they are
involved in the daily care of their clients. Therefore, an interest should be
taken in the different leisure pursuits which promote muscle movement,
bone and joint mobility ensuring that exercise can be fun and relaxing as well
as therapeutic.

Other aspects of exercise and mobility are discussed in the chapters
which relate to the different client groups (Chapters 6–10).

Environment

It is important for a care provider to create a safe and comfortable environment for clients. If a room, residential home, day centre, day nursery or
classroom is made to look interesting, homely and welcoming, it will create a
sense of well-being for both client and carer.

There are some basic principles which apply to most environments,
such as:

- pleasant decorations with flowers, plants and pictures
- windows which can be opened so that the room can be aired regularly.
  They also enable the sun to shine into the room
- colourful curtains and blinds
- basic furniture such as comfortable seating, sufficient chairs, tables or
  beds for the number of service users
- sufficient space between chairs and tables. Service users should have some
  personal space to be able to move position without encroaching on the
  space of others
- access for wheelchairs
- non-slip floor covering or carpeting
- Health and Safety inspection, such as a risk assessment, to ensure the
  environment is safe and has no area or equipment which may be a hazard
  to the client
- remembering that clients have different tastes and ideas in interior decoration and design.

EMOTIONAL NEEDS

Emotional needs of individuals are closely associated with their health and well-being and, according to Maslow these needs relate to:

- *survival* – basic/physiological needs: the need to live, and to be supported to live
- *security* – safety needs: the need to feel secure and safe from harm
- *belonging* – social and love needs: the need to be accepted by others, i.e. to feel loved and wanted
- *prestige* – esteem needs: the need to have talents and abilities recognised in a positive way, i.e. to have a sense of achievement
- *fulfilment* – self-actualisation needs: the need to enjoy life's challenges, to lead a satisfying and happy life.

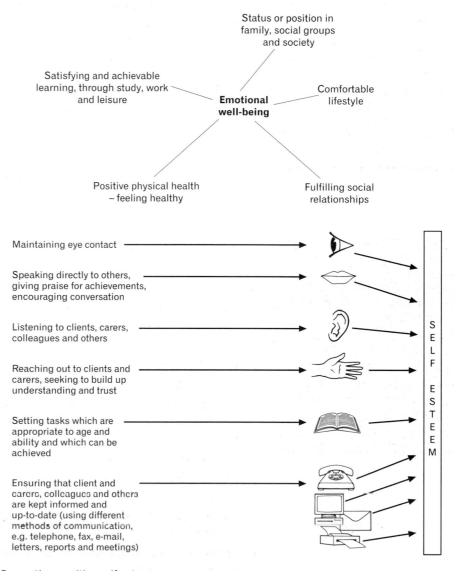

Promoting positive self-esteem

In addition, individuals have a need to feel that they can be physically close in an intimate sexual relationship with another person. Sexuality is an important feature of the way that individuals view themselves and how they relate to themselves and to others.

Carers who are aware of a client's emotional needs will also recognise that how a person views themself is an important part of their **self-concept**. Self-concept includes a person's self-esteem and self-image. There are different ways in which an individual relates to the feelings that they have about their bodies, height, weight and looks. These are interpreted and linked through a person's thinking and emotional feelings. Therefore praise and encouragement can be a major factor in promoting a positive self-esteem and view of self.

CASE STUDY

George

George is drawing a picture. He thinks his picture will make his mother say 'well done' as she usually does. He feels a real sense of achievement about his drawing. Harry comes up to him and says 'What's that scribble?'
George immediately feels that his picture is not very good and he responds by screwing up his piece of paper and running away.

1   What are the issues involved here?

2   How should carers react in this situation?

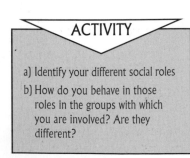

KEY POINT

A person's social development will reflect the way in which they relate to other individuals, groups and the different social agencies such as family, school, work and the community in which they live.

ACTIVITY

a) Identify your different social roles
b) How do you behave in those roles in the groups with which you are involved? Are they different?

SOCIAL NEEDS

Social needs cover the ways in which individuals are able to relate to each other. This involves the need for friends and to be part of groups, to be accepted by others and to be able to fit in without feeling awkward and shy. In addition to this, it is important to be able to make conversation, make friends with others, be popular with their peers and to behave in a way which is appropriate to them. In fact, the **social role** which they adopt, when they meet others as individuals or groups, is a feature of their social relationships.

A social role is a person's position in society which requires them to act in particular ways. People have to carry out different roles in society. A woman may be a wife, mother, daughter and nurse. In some situations, individuals dress according to the role they have. For example, the woman who is a nurse will wear different clothes for work and for home.

Communication and interpersonal relationships are very important to individuals and to their social roles.

Once in a care setting, a client may have to change their social role, and this will affect their self-concept. Clients who have been very independent may find it difficult to adjust to being dependent.

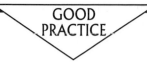

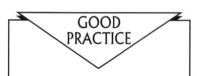
CASE STUDY

Martin and Gill

Martin and Gill are active 65-year-olds. They are enjoying their retirement and are involved in a variety of activities, such as ballroom dancing, skittles, drama club and walking holidays. One day Martin falls off a ladder. He is taken to hospital with two broken legs.

What are the key issues involved with regard to Martin's changing social role?

From this case study we learn that the individual social role is a valuable part of a person's identity. However, being in a group where individuals can meet together, share joint interests and activities, can be very much a part of leisure roles. Having friends and sharing activities is often a relaxing part of life. Weekends, or days off, enable people to relax and take time for themselves.

Recreation needs

Providing for a client's recreation needs – the way a person wishes to spend their leisure time – is an active way of meeting social needs. Recreation:

- provides interest leading to new hobbies and different leisure pursuits
- provides further opportunities for social contact
- gives pleasure and can be a satisfying experience.

Recreation programmes in different care settings can include creative and craft activities, such as art, collage, drama, dress-making, flower arranging, keep fit, or interest groups which involve day trips, short breaks or holidays visiting historical places of interest.

KEY POINTS

In homes and day hospitals care workers often make the mistake of offering group activities and expecting everyone to join in. Consider setting up a number of small groups and offering individual activities. This will help carers meet differing care needs. The charity Counsel and Care produce two useful booklets about activities:

- **Not Only Bingo** (1990) – a study of good practice in providing leisure activities for older people. Many of the ideas outlined can be adapted to other client groups
- **Leisure, Later Life and Homes** (1995) – information and ideas for leisure activities in homes.

These booklets point out that activities should be tailored to individual needs and wishes.

INTELLECTUAL AND COGNITIVE NEEDS

Intellectual and cognitive needs of individuals reflect the learning, problem-solving, memory, thinking and understanding processes in the human brain.

The brain can be regarded as a large computer centre where information is stored, problems are solved, messages are retained, and messages are sent out using different sources, such as language. It is interesting to note that the mind, behaviour and the personality depend on the interaction between the brain and the body.

A baby's skills and responses have to be learned. As she grows and develops every movement supplies feedback to the brain. She will learn through the different sensory experiences during the first few months of life. What she sees, hears, touches, tastes and smells will create the relevant perceptions of the world around her. These are retained by the brain for future use.

Language development is closely linked to intellectual and cognitive development and provides the way in which individuals communicate. It is a structured set of sounds which is associated with thought and memory. When people talk to each other, they use their thought processes to reason and problem-solve as they listen to what is being said. As they understand the words being said, they are able to respond and answer. This is an important aspect of communication, essential for meeting social needs, as already discussed on page 44.

Learning needs

Intellectual and cognitive skills are linked to the learning needs of individuals. In a child's early years the desire to create, imagine, understand, problem-solve, reason and concentrate on many different tasks and activities should be encouraged and developed through the family, playgroups, nursery classes and school. However, sometimes, the learning and development of intellectual and cognitive needs are slowed down or interrupted, for example:

- *at birth*, when a baby is born with a congenital disability or birth injury
- as a result of *sensory impairments*, such as visual or hearing impairments
- as a result of an *accident or injury* which affects the brain, such as head injuries and strokes
- by *disease* which affects memory and is progressive, such as Alzheimer's disease (Alzheimer's more commonly affects older people)
- as a result of *disorders to the brain*, such as a brain tumour which needs surgery – parts of the brain may be removed with the tumour, therefore reducing cognitive functioning
- as a result of *drugs* – side effects can cause concentration loss.

A learning need may be evident before a child begins school or become evident during their school life, such as dyslexia.

Whatever the learning need which has developed, it affects the view that a person has of the world around them. At times the world can seem frightening, especially for those who have previously been in control of faculties such as the ability to think and speak. For example, a client may have had a stroke which affects their speech. They may find their jumbled thoughts and their lack of speech disturbing and distressing. The early days after a stroke are very important in terms of support and sensitive care. It is distressing for close family and friends who have to learn to cope with the discomfort and frustration of their loved one.

Clients with learning or physical disabilities have learning needs which should be recognised and reinforced with loving, encouraging and supportive care. This is augmented by the carer giving clients the incentive to achieve, however small or simple the task. This enables clients to feel more positive about themselves and to come to terms with their disability.

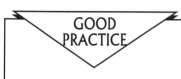

GOOD PRACTICE

In meeting the learning requirements of clients, carers can:

- design tasks and activities to stimulate thinking, problem-solving, reasoning, memory and language. This may involve breaking a task down into smaller steps so that the client can achieve success. This is explained in more depth in Chapter 5 page 55
- modify and adapt equipment so that it can be used by clients with limited manipulative or fine motor skills
- match the activity with the learning need
- use bright, colourful objects, sounds and textures to promote sight, sound and touch
- ensure that the environment is conducive to the needs of the client. Some centres have sensory rooms where clients can lie or sit on cushions and look at different lights and movement in the room
- develop an understanding of the various learning needs of the clients in the different care settings.

What then are the main requirements for a carer working with a client who has a learning need or limited intellectual and cognitive development? It is important to remind ourselves of the tools for learning in the first years of life, i.e. learning by observation, doing and association.

ROLE PLAY | **Jimmy**

In order to understand the learning needs of clients, role-play the following situation.

Jimmy is 20 years old, has Down's syndrome and lives with his mother and father in a large house in the country. He wants to move away from home and to live in a flat with two friends, Linda and Brian, whom he met at the local day centre.

In groups, act out the parts of Jimmy, his parents and his two friends.

- Identify the needs of Jimmy.
- Explore the concerns of the parents.
- Work through the different learning issues which arise in this situation.
- What strategies can be introduced by the social worker to support Jimmy?

Supporting a client's learning can be a rewarding experience for a carer. To be part of a caring process which encourages and supports a client's sense of understanding and knowledge of the world around them, and then to see them respond in their own individual way, is an aspect of caring which should always be cherished by both the carer and their clients.

CULTURAL NEEDS

The various cultures which make up modern-day society bring into sharper focus the different beliefs, values, customs and lifestyles which are involved. It is important that carers make themselves familiar with the customs involved in caring for *all* clients.

People with the same ethnic origin may have very different cultures. For example, a person who is African-Caribbean may have been raised in the USA, the UK or the West Indies. Cultural needs are not only dependent on a person's ethnic needs, but also on a person's upbringing, values and religion.

There are certain aspects of culture which affect the care needs of individuals, including:

- *Diet*, for example:
  - Hindus consider cows sacred and do not eat beef. Some are vegetarian.
  - Muslims consider pigs to be unclean and do not eat pork. Strict Muslims only eat *halal* meat – this means that the animal has been slaughtered in a certain way.
  - Jews consider pork or shellfish unclean and do not eat them. Strict Jews follow a *kosher* diet and have separate areas in the kitchen for preparing meat and milk dishes. Separate crockery is also used for

meat and milk dishes. Meat and milk are not eaten together or at the same meal.
- Parsees do not have any dietary restrictions.
- Buddhists often follow a vegan diet and avoid all animal products.
- *Dress*, for example:
  - Hindus often wear traditional dress, such as saris.
  - Muslim men do not wear gold. They may wear traditional or western clothing. Muslim women may wear traditional or western dress. Most Muslim women tend to dress modestly and keep their upper arms covered. Some women prefer to wear long skirts, few would wear skirts shorter than knee length.
  - Jewish men may wear the traditional skull cap (kippah) on the crown.
  - Parsees wear a sacred thread tied around the waist and a white cotton undershirt. The sacred thread is never removed. The undershirt is washed by hand, usually by a member of the family.
- *Lifestyle*, for example:
  - Hindu culture is based on a caste system and a person is born into a particular caste, from which they cannot move. Their lifestyle is based on their caste.
  - Muslims consider the left hand to be unclean. Offering anything with the left hand is considered a grave insult. Left-handed care workers should make sure they offer food, medication, etc. with their right hands. Muslim women do not allow people other than their husband and other women to see them naked. Most Muslim women would not wish to have a male care worker.
- *Religion* – see the next section.

Note that the above are only examples. Carers and care workers need to make themselves aware of the cultural practices of their individual clients. This will help them to meet their cultural needs, and aid the care relationship.

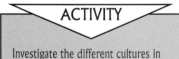

ACTIVITY

Investigate the different cultures in your own local community. Research the differences in terms of diet, lifestyle and religion.

SPIRITUAL NEEDS

People of all faiths have spiritual needs. People with care needs can find it difficult to attend their place of worship. Often care workers suggest that a minister visits the person at home. However, many people with care needs find this less satisfying than worshipping with others. They feel that only by visiting a place of worship can they enjoy the music, atmosphere and social aspects of worshipping. Ministers of all faiths can usually arrange for volunteers to take the person to the place of worship. This enables the person to participate fully and meets their spiritual needs.

Religious celebrations

Every faith has special celebrations associated with it, for example:

- Hindus celebrate Diwali
- Muslims observe Ramadan, a time of fasting and reflection. They celebrate its end with Eid, a time of festivities

Within every individual there is a spiritual dimension and, therefore, a spiritual need, but this is not always a religious one. The sense of spirituality covers the whole range of a person's life experience. How they relate to these experiences has a considerable influence upon them. This will vary according to a person's lifestyle, beliefs, values, culture and social background.

KEY TERMS

You need to know the meaning of the following words and phrases. Go back through the chapter to make sure that you understand them.

cultural needs
culture
emotional needs
healthy diet
holistic care
intellectual and cognitive
    needs
physical needs
self-concept
social needs
social role
spiritual needs

- Jews celebrate the Passover. They observe the Sabbath every Saturday with a special celebration, usually with their family.
- Christians celebrate Christ's birth at Christmas, and his resurrection at Easter.

Meeting spiritual needs

Carers and care workers need to make themselves aware of the religious practices of their individual clients. This will help them to meet their spiritual needs, and aid the care relationship.

Care workers can help a person meet spiritual needs by recognising these needs and offering assistance if required. For example:

- A Catholic may wish to avoid meat on Fridays or fast days.
- A Muslim may require help to wash before prayer.
- A Jew may require help to prepare to observe the Sabbath.

Enabling a person to meet spiritual needs can make a real difference to that person's quality of life.

In caring for others it is important to understand that spiritual needs are influenced by the whole range of a person's life, personal, cultural and spiritual experiences. It should be remembered that these experiences are unique to each individual, and therefore spiritual needs will differ accordingly.

Aspects of care

This chapter focuses on issues that are important to all individuals who are involved in caring for others. The key topics covered in this chapter are:

- Care planning
- Supporting a client with living needs
- Problems in care relationships
- Caring for the carer
- Coping with the stress of caring.

While the chapters in Part 2 explore aspects which arise in the different client groups, this chapter will address some of the issues which relate to care practice in general.

Supporting a client with daily living needs and being able to assess those needs was discussed at the end of Chapter 1 and identified as an important part of modern-day caring. Needs and how to meet them were discussed in detail in Chapter 4. It is now important to look at how a client's needs are determined and met by **care planning**.

CARE PLANNING

Care planning is the process of **assessment** of a client's needs and agreeing the care, treatment or therapy between professional carers and their clients, following assessment. The resulting plan of care is called the **care plan**.

Care planning follows a number of stages (see the care planning cycle diagram opposite).

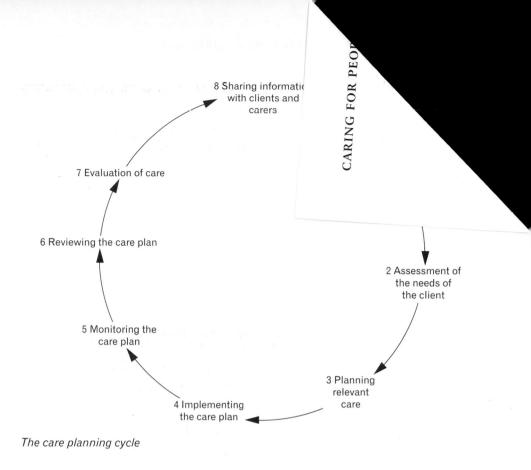

The care planning cycle

Assessment

Assessment is the process of defining the needs of an individual client. Following the NHS and Community Care Act in 1990, assessment and management of care was confirmed as a principle requirement to be addressed by local authorities in the care of their clients. Thus social service departments have a legal duty to assess a client's needs.

There are two main types of assessment:

- *self assessment*, in which a client monitors and evaluates their own views of their abilities and their care needs
- *observation*, in which a carer or care worker watches the client carrying out a task. Following this observation the carer can discuss the different needs which may have arisen from the task.

Whenever assessment takes place, a checklist is drawn up to agree with the client that the relevant areas have been addressed. The assessment checklist includes the following questions (from Clark, Sachs and Ford, 1995).

- Has the assessment been negotiated with the potential client? Is the client aware that they are being assessed or do they think the discussion is an informal one? Has the assessor explained their role and why they are there?
- Has the appropriate setting for the assessment been chosen? It is important that both the assessor and the client are comfortable and at ease.

- Have the client and the carer been **empowered** to take part in the process, taking into account their ethnic, cultural or communication needs?
- Does the client have access to someone to act as a advocate, i.e. someone who can speak on their behalf and represent their interests?
- Have any differing perceptions of need been clarified and, if so, have they been recorded?
- Does the client know if they are eligible for the service they have requested?
- Have the client's needs been prioritised and have objectives been set for each of those needs?
- Has the client seen and agreed the written record of assessment?
- Does the client know when they may request reassessment?
- Do they understand how to complain if dissatisfied?
- Does the client know that they may decline assistance if they wish to do so unless there is statutory invention?

Assessment is a normal part of the care process. Most carers and care workers assess and monitor those in their care on a regular basis. Assessment of needs allows carers to be involved in prioritising care with the client.

Different organisations assess clients and service users at different levels. For example, social care assessment can involve a number of levels, to enable specialist and complex assessments to be targeted to those clients and their families who need them most.

Care plans

Functions of a care plan
A care plan:

- enables family and friends to be involved in how the plan is implemented
- allows the client to be involved in their care requirements
- enables health and social care workers to work together as a multi-disciplinary team to plan, implement and deliver care
- keeps the client informed of their care
- means that the client is regularly monitored, reviewed and evaluated.

Setting up a care plan
Setting up a care plan is an important aspect of a professional carer's work. Collaboration with other services is essential so that the provision of a cost-effective package of care services can be set up to meet the client's needs. It involves:

- the client
- the client's family
- carers (formal and informal) and their different roles and responsibilities
- the care manager/assessor (see below)
- the assessor

- any agencies or support groups who may work together or may collaborate in meeting the needs of the client.

Care management describes the strategy for co-ordinating and reviewing the care plan. This is usually the task of the care manager who will co-ordinate services to meet the care requirements of the client within the determined criteria and budget. The care manager is responsible for assessment, monitoring and reviewing.

Care plans may be:

- developed by one professional, for example a care manager, nurse or social worker
- jointly devised by a multi-disciplinary or multi-professional team; for example, a multi-disciplinary team responsible for developing a care plan for a client with physical disabilities might include the person's GP, social worker, occupational therapist, speech therapist and care manager
- developed by the client themselves, working with the appropriate health and social care professionals. This is an important aspect of setting up a care plan as it enables the client to take control of their own planning.

The results of the assessment and the care plan should be confirmed in writing or in accessible format to both the client and the carer.

CASE STUDY

John

John is an older man who suffers from confusion. He has lived alone for many years in a large house. He has managed to cope on his own until his recent bout of flu. Since his illness, he has become more confused. Recently, he fell down the stairs and broke his arm. He has no close relatives living nearby. He is finding looking after himself and the house difficult.

1 A care planning meeting has been set up for John. How would you make sure that John's views are represented?

2 Set up a care plan for John, describing how many people will be involved in his care.

SUPPORTING A CLIENT WITH LIVING NEEDS

In Chapter 4, the activities of daily living were identified. Living needs form the basis for these. Supporting living needs is a means whereby carers can assist a person in their care to maintain their daily lives. This process is often written into the care plan.

A client may be supported by their carer or care worker to:

- *be able to choose a lifestyle and to flourish,* i.e. maintain a good quality of life, which includes an adequate and healthy diet, leisure activities and pleasant environment

- *be independent*, i.e. to make decisions and to feel a sense of achievement
- *feel accepted*, i.e. to have a sense of belonging
- *be able to speak*, i.e. to be listened to and to feel that what they are saying has value
- *be able to move around*, i.e. to be mobile and to go places
- *retain their identity*, i.e. which includes sexual, physical, spiritual and cultural aspects
- *have personal space*, i.e. privacy
- *be financially secure, independent*, i.e. to have a home of their own and money to spend.

Factors which increase the need for support

There are various factors that increase the support a client may require from a carer or care worker. These are:

- *physical factors*, such as a disease, disorder or dysfunction which may have damaged parts of the body. This means that the body is unable to work normally in order to achieve body movement. For example, damage to the spinal cord can lead to paralysis which affects a person's mobility and movement
- *psychological factors*, such as a disease, disorder or dysfunction which may affect the mental health of a person. For example, a person suffering with dementia may need help and support with personal hygiene and toileting
- *intellectual factors*, such as a disease, disorder and dysfunction which affects the problem-solving and learning processes in the brain. For example, a person with Down's syndrome may need to be taught different skills to maintain their daily living
- *environmental factors*, such as poverty, inadequate housing and poor living conditions which may reduce the ways in which a person can meet their living needs and may disrupt the necessary activity of **living skills**.

There are many situations in which a carer or care worker may be required to teach a client or a person in their care a living skill – a skill that will enable them to carry out daily activities in order to maintain their lifestyle. These can range from supporting a client's mobility, showing them how to walk with a walking aid, helping the client who is recovering from a stroke to make a cup of tea, or teaching hygiene routines to a client with a learning disability.

There are different types of living skill:

- *self-help skills*, such as dressing, washing, bathing
- *motor skills*: gross motor skills, such as walking, running, and fine motor skills, such as picking up objects
- *communication skills*, such as reinforcing speech and language
- *social skills*, such as encouraging clients to meet with others, building relationships.

Teaching a living skill

Care planning has an important role to play in identifying the skills that may need to be taught. Once identified, there is a framework that the care and care worker can use to teach a skill and support the client. The framework is:

- *identification of the skill* – which task is to be learned

- *task analysis* – can the skill be broken down into a number of simpler tasks which can be tackled one at a time?

- *demonstration of the skill* – the carer shows how the task is carried out and makes sure that the client understands

- *opportunities for skill practice* – setting up a programme where the task can be practised on a regular basis

- *monitoring of the skill* – the skill is observed by the carer at regular intervals and assessed (observing how the client is coping, discussing positive aspects and exploring areas of concern). The carer should be giving the client positive encouragement and praise at every stage of the process

- *evaluation and review* – the learning of the skill is assessed as part of the care plan evaluation and review.

These steps should be carried out with the permission of the client or their **advocate**.

Once the skill has been mastered it may be necessary to introduce another skill. The monitoring, review and evaluation of the care plan ensures that the quality of care which supports the client reinforces their autonomy, independence, access, rights and choices.

CASE STUDY

Mr Jones

Mr Jones is 89 years old. His wife has died recently and Mr Jones now lives alone. After discussion with him about his needs and the services available to meet those needs, it was decided that as part of his care plan, Mr Jones should be taught to cook simple meals for himself.

As his care worker:

1 How would you help Mr Jones?

2 Use the framework for teaching a skill to design a programme for Mr Jones.

PROBLEMS IN CARE RELATIONSHIPS

The development of a professional care relationship between client and care worker is at the heart of caring (see Chapter 1). It is vital to the success of the service that these relationships are optimised.

Lack of attention to the care relationship means not just failure to provide an effective service, but possibly considerable damage and distress to clients. Nevertheless, there are many common problems that arise in caring relationships, and it is useful to be aware of them in case they occur. They include the following.

Lack of self-awareness

Not all relationships go smoothly. This is sometimes due to the care worker's lack of self-awareness in some areas. This is the sort of issue where regular supervision is useful, and which needs to be supported with continued training.

Care workers have a professional obligation to strive continuously to develop their awareness and skills. There is a responsibility on the part of the agency that employs them to ensure this happens through the provision of supervision and further training.

Loss of respect for the client

The importance of acceptance of the client in a care relationship cannot be stressed enough. This is based on the philosophical conviction that every person has innate dignity and worth.

Sometimes, however, the client may behave in ways, or express beliefs or feelings, which may be reprehensible to the carer. Only a skilled care worker can successfully manage such a dilemma. When the care worker experiences difficulty with this, supervision should be urgently sought.

Over-identification

Sometimes the care worker feels very strongly about the difficulties a client is experiencing. Perhaps the care worker has had personal experience of similar problems. Commonly, this may involve attitudes toward authority. The carer soon starts to respond to his or her own needs, rather than to those of the client. Here, too, diligence is required, and supervision should be urgently sought.

The feeling of power

Sometimes the care worker will assume that, because he or she has the responsibility of care, this is somehow a statement of competence, which is interpreted as a sign of personal adequacy or superiority.

The powerlessness of the client can provide a real sense of control on the part of the care worker. When things go well, the care worker takes the credit. However, when things go badly, the client is often blamed. It is important to remember that clients do not often share the freedoms that the care worker may have. The care worker may withdraw from the relationship, while the client is dependent on it. Examples of withdrawal include changing jobs or gaining promotion.

This sort of problem is quite serious, and is often not just the fault of the individual care worker, but of the whole culture of the care setting. To avoid such a problem developing, vigilance is required by both care workers and managers.

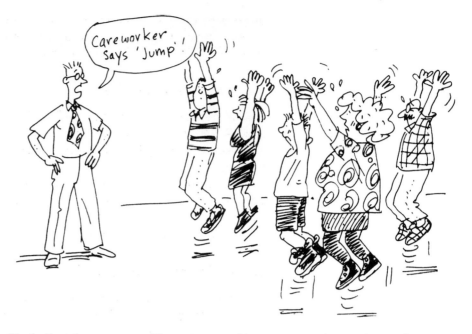

The feeling of power – one of the common problems a care worker must recognise

Insincerity

Insincerity is often the problem of the more seasoned care worker, who has given a great deal emotionally, with seemingly little reward. Most care workers seek moral, rather than financial, rewards and the feedback they require to continue to motivate them is often lacking. Care workers who are insincere are in danger not of just ceasing to care, but of actually rejecting their clients.

Ruthlessness and expediency

Care workers often face emotional bombardment, and develop high levels of stress. In this condition, the care worker cannot thoughtfully monitor his or her relationship with the client. Remember, the professional care relationship is controlled – it has boundaries. Under stress, however, these boundaries may be overstepped. Workers respond by doing what is most expedient – they take the easiest course. This can result in inappropriate ruthlessness, where clients' feelings are not considered. The recognition of stress in care work is important, page 61 (Clarke, Sachs and Ford, 1995).

ROLE PLAY   Claire

In groups of three, role-play the following situation and try to find a resolution to the problem. The parts to be taken are:
- you (care assistant)
- Claire
- the care manager.

You work as a care assistant. Your job is to help a 35-year-old woman called Claire. Claire lives in a ground floor flat which is adapted for a wheelchair user. She is paraplegic, i.e. paralysed from the waist down. She has a 6-year-old daughter called Courtney. Claire needs 24-hour care. The care manager has arranged a meeting with Claire because Claire has said that you are 'not very caring' and that she feels you do not like her.
- Determine Claire's care needs in this situation.
- What has occurred in the care relationship?
- How can the difficulties be resolved?

Guidelines and codes of conduct

There are differences between the roles of the formal and informal carer. The formal carer is guided by the policies and procedures of the organisation which employs them and by the body that regulates the profession of which they are a part. Some regulatory guidelines that affect the work of formal carers are to be found in:

- Appendix 1A: Code of Professional Conduct for Nurses
- Appendix 1B: Code of Professional Conduct for Social Workers
- Chapter 3, page 23, the Care Value Base.

Informal carers by the very nature of their work, have no obvious, formal frameworks to guide the caring that they do. This can be a cause of concern for some informal carers – they have no professional boundaries to work within, but they feel that they do have a 'duty to care'. The burden of caring can often leave them stressed, isolated and alone.

CASE STUDY

David and Jean

David and Jean have been married for 20 years. They have two teenage boys, aged 14 and 16, who are still at school. David has been diagnosed with terminal cancer and has had to give up work because of medical treatment which has left him weak. Jean is constantly on the move, trying to manage her job and hold the family together. There are times she feels so exhausted but what can she do?

1 List the different pressures on Jean.

2 Devise a strategy of support for Jean.

CARING FOR THE CARERS

Caring for the carers is a term which indicates an awareness of the needs of those who care for others in a variety of settings. In the past ten years there has been a growing awareness of the needs of those who care for relatives, friends and neighbours on a long-term and often full-time basis. Those issues which relate mainly to informal carers have been identified in the Carers Recognition and Services Act 1995 and in the philosophy which guides the Carers National Association.

The needs of informal carers

The role of informal carer, and the impact that providing unpaid care for a relative or friend can have, has become a subject of concern over the last 20 years. It is now acknowledged that informal carers have a tremendous burden to carry in caring for their loved ones, friends or relatives.

This concern has gradually led to pressure being imposed on the Government to identify ways of helping and supporting informal carers. Pat Young (1985) identifies the provision of informal care as a key element of community care. In her discussion of this aspect of community care, she uses research to offer some interesting insights on who informal carers are and how caring affects them. The findings of the study included the following.

- The people whom informal carers care for are generally their own relatives.
- Women are much more likely to provide informal care than men.
- Men who do provide informal care generally care for wives. Women care for a much broader range of relatives.
- Informal carers often receive little support from other family members.
- Caring tends to dominate the informal carer's life.

According to research carried out by the King's Fund Informal Caring Programme in 1995, there are approximately six million informal carers in the UK today. Most of these people care for a relative or friend who is old or ill. Some experience stress and exhaustion. Following this research, a ten-point plan was drawn up with regard to carers' needs. It was proposed that carers should receive the following.

1   Recognition of their contribution and of their needs as individuals in their own right.
2   Services tailored to their individual circumstances, needs and views, through discussions at the time help is being planned.
3   Services which reflect an awareness of differing racial, cultural and religious backgrounds and values, equally accessible to carers of every race and ethnic origin.
4   Opportunities, both for short spells (an afternoon) and for longer periods (a week or more), to relax and have time to themselves.
5   Practical help to lighten the tasks of caring, including domestic help, home adaptations, incontinence services and support with transport.
6   Someone to talk to about their own emotional needs, at the outset of caring, while they are caring and when the caring task is over.

7   Information about available benefits and services as well as how to cope with the particular condition of the person being cared for.

8   An income which covers the cost of caring and which does not preclude carers taking employment or sharing care with other people.

9   Opportunities to explore alternatives to family care, both for the immediate and long-term future.

10   Services designed through consultation with carers, at all levels of policy planning. (King's Fund, 1995)

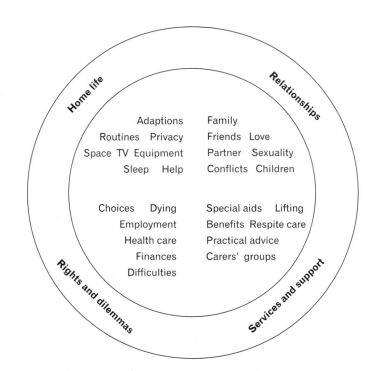

The needs of the informal carer (Brown and Bassett, 1996)

Given the large and important contribution that informal carers make, it is arguable that formal care services should be designed in consultation with them to ensure that their needs can also be met. This idea was endorsed by a range of national carer support groups including the Carers National Association, Crossroads Care and the National Schizophrenia Fellowship (King's Fund, 1995). There are now a number of pieces of legislation which include provisions aimed at supporting informal carers.

Support groups for informal carers

There are various locally organised support groups in the UK. Many of these exist to meet the needs of informal carers (see the diagram opposite). One of the key national organisations that provides a range of services, including lobbying the Government, on behalf of informal carers is the Carers National Association (CNA). It has four aims:

- to encourage informal carers to recognise their own needs
- to develop appropriate advice for informal carers
- to provide information for informal carers
- to bring the needs of informal carers to the attention of the Government and those involved in policy-making.

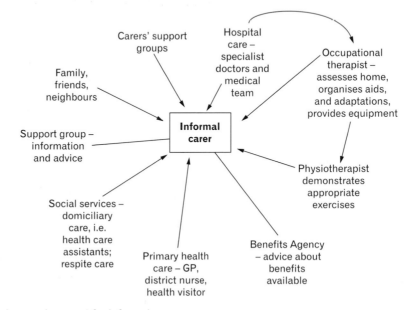

Services and support for informal carers

COPING WITH THE STRESS OF CARING

Caring for others is a stressful business. Working with people, looking after their individual and different needs, helping them to feel better, all make demands on an individual's physical, emotional and intellectual resources and social time. Often people who undertake demanding care roles find themselves so busy caring for others that they forget about their own needs and experience forms of **stress** that are destructive and damaging to them as individuals and as carers.

Part of coping with caring involves identifying one's own needs, and working towards meeting these needs. By doing so carers and care workers are in a better position to seek the appropriate and necessary support, to which they are entitled.

Stress

Stress is a commonly used term. Most people will say that they suffer from stress at certain times in their lives. Stress is unwelcome pressure and the resultant feeling of being unable to cope with demands on one's time and abilities. It is a common feature of care relationships because of the major physical, emotional and psychological demands that caring makes on the carer.

Stress levels typically build up when carers:

- feel that they do not meet the expectations of their clients or the people they are helping
- think that they do not meet the expectation of their managers
- have to work with insufficient resources in terms of finance, equipment, environment and time
- feel that there are difficult professional relationships which are caused by a lack of communication
- find that the continuous and demanding role of caring does not always fulfil the needs of the clients, for example, the client may be dying or may be readmitted to hospital.

Informal carers also experience high levels of stress because of the immense changes that occur in their relationships and in their daily lives when they take on the role of caring for a relative or friend at home.

Researchers have come up with a league table of stressful situations and have given each situation a stress rating (see Table 5.1).

Stress factor	Rating	Stress factor	Rating
Death of a spouse or partner	100	Change in responsibilities at work	29
Divorce	73	Son or daughter leaving home	29
Marital separation	65	Trouble with in-laws	29
Jail term	63	Outstanding personal achievement	28
Death of close family member	63	Wife or female partner begins or stops work	26
Personal injury or illness	53	Begin or end school	26
Marriage	50	Change in living conditions	25
Fired at work	47	Revision of personal habits	24
Made redundant	45	Trouble with boss at work	23
Marital reconciliation	45	Change in work hours or conditions	23
Retirement	45	Change in residence	20
Pregnancy	40	Change in school	20
Change of health of family member	39	Change in recreation	19
Sex difficulties	39	Change in religious activities	19
Gain of new family member	39	Change in social activities	18
Business readjustment	39	Mortgage or loans less than £10,000*	17
Change in financial state	38	Change in sleeping habits	16
Death of close friend	37	Change in number of family get-togethers	15
Change to a different line of work	36	Change in eating habits	15
Change in number of arguments with spouse or partner	35	Holiday	15
Mortgage over £10,000*	31	Minor violation of the law	11
Foreclosure of mortgage or loan	30	*[1967 figures]	

Table 5.1 Stress ratings (Holmes and Rahe, 1967)

Signs of stress

As a carer and care worker it is vital to be aware of the key signs of stress and **burn-out**. It is also important that carers and care workers respond appropriately to potential stress by using **stress management** (see page 65).

The first signs of stress can be seen in an individual's:

- *sleep pattern* – inability to sleep, waking up early
- *eating pattern* – loss of appetite or overeating or eating very quickly
- *increased intake of alcohol, coffee and tea* – drinking tea and coffee to produce more energy. Increasing intake of alcohol to relax and forget
- *smoking* – smoking more cigarettes in an effort to feel more relaxed
- *sexual behaviour* – after giving so much of the emotional self, there is a need to feel close and sexually intimate, or to view the sexual relationship as just one more demand and a chore
- *mood and behaviour changes* – trying to be happy when with others, but feeling drained and depressed when alone. Becoming withdrawn and isolated from others.

The physical effects of short-term and long-term stress are shown in the diagrams below and on page 64.

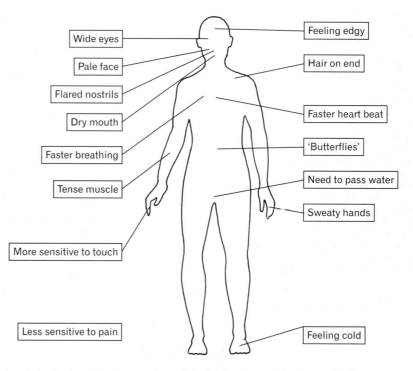

The physical effects of short-term stress (Clarke, Sachs and Waltham, 1994)

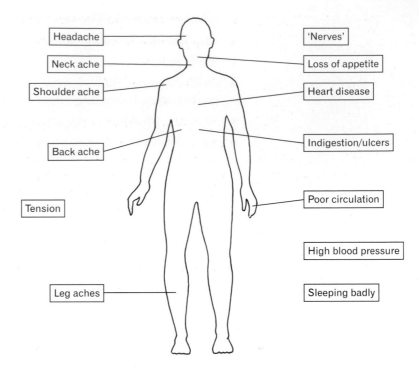

The physical effects of long-term stress (Clarke, Sachs and Waltham, 1994)

The experience of burn-out

If stress is not managed, it can damage a carer's health or lead to burn-out – continuous feelings of exhaustion, tension and disillusionment, negative attitudes to work. There are several indicators which show a carer that the stress they are experiencing is becoming something deeper and may lead to burn-out. These include (Moonie *et al.*, 1995):

- high resistance to work every day (not wanting to go there, to be there or do the work)
- suspicion and fear of other people
- a sense of failure
- feelings of anger, resentment and negativity to clients and colleagues
- feelings of guilt and blame towards oneself and others
- isolation and withdrawal
- feeling tired and exhausted all day
- stereotyping clients and others
- inability to listen to other people
- poor sleep patterns

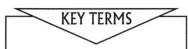

- frequent colds and illnesses leading to time off work
- frequent headaches and stomach upsets
- alcohol abuse
- conflict with others
- rigid thinking.

Carers are highly likely to face stressful situations on a regular basis because the nature of the work they do involves close contact, often for long periods of time, with people in distress and individuals with unresolved problems. This can lead to physical, emotional and psychological exhaustion in the carer and care worker. Where stress is a regular, inevitable part of an individual's daily life, stress management strategies should be explored and used.

Stress management

When symptoms of stress begin to occur it may be helpful to deal with these initial signs by reviewing the following.

- *Diet* – Look at your dietary intake. Is it healthy, containing the right foods, or does it consist of junk food and take-aways?
- *Discussion* – Are you able to discuss your difficulties and problems? Can a friend or member of the family help by listening?
- *Exercise* – Do you take opportunities for exercise? Exercise can help to lower blood pressure.
- *Take time off* – Are you making time for some rest, relaxation and personal space?

If high levels of stress do not respond to management through diet, talking, exercise or time off, then there are also a number of individual stress control/relaxation methods that can be used. These include counselling, behaviour therapy, psychotherapy, yoga and massage, and other alternative therapies.

PART 2

THE CLIENT GROUPS

Part 2 explores the different aspects of caring discussed in Part 1 in the context of the client groups across the lifespan. The chapters are:

6 ▷ *Caring for babies*

7 ▷ *Caring for children*

8 ▷ *Caring for adolescents*

9 ▷ *Caring for adults*

10 ▷ *Caring for older people*

Each chapter discusses the following aspects for each client group:
- Growth and development
- Basic needs
- Care issues
- Life events
- Special and additional needs
- Sources of support.

In order to develop a clearer understanding of the psycho-social needs for the development of the different client groups, Erikson's model of psycho-social development (see the table on page 68) is referred to in each chapter.

Stage	Approximate age range	Developmental stages	Personality features	Negative aspects
1	0–1½ years	Basic trust versus mistrust	Sense of hope and safety	Insecurity, anxiety
2	1½–3 years	Self-control versus shame and doubt	Learning self-control and independence	Dependent and unable to control events
3	3–7 years	Initiative versus guilt	Direction and purpose in life	Lack of self-esteem
4	6–15 years	Industry versus inferiority	Building skills competence and positive self-esteem	Feels inferior and lacks confidence
5	13–21 years	Identity versus role confusion	A developing sense of self confidence and security	No direction in life. Negative self-esteem
6	18–30 years	Intimacy versus isolation	Building relationships, loving commitment	Unable to build relationships
7	20s–60s	Generativity versus stagnation	Caring for others – reaching out in the community	Introverted – looking inwards – concerned with self
8	Later life	Ego-integrity versus despair	Sense of meaning to life	Loss of sense of achievement

Erikson's model of psycho-social development (Erikson, 1963)

The activities in the following chapters provide opportunities to apply different skills in a variety of situations.

Caring for babies

PREVIEW

Knowledge of the skills needed to meet babies' individual needs is vital in the provision of their care in a variety of care settings. These settings demand different skills and strategies of care. This chapter will enable you to develop your understanding of:
- Growth and development
- Basic needs
- Care issues
- Life events
- Special and additional needs
- Sources of support.

When they are born, human babies are helpless. But they do have various body systems which work independently and support their physical development. These include life-supporting body activities such as breathing, response to light and sound, kidney, liver and heart functions. Supporting a baby's development of these systems is central to their care.

In addition to this, the holistic approach to caring caters for other aspects of a baby's development, such as intellectual and cognitive, social and emotional well-being

GROWTH AND DEVELOPMENT

Babies progress through a number of stages, or milestones of growth and development, during the early years of their lives. They grow at a rapid rate, physically, emotionally, socially, intellectually and in other ways such as in language development.

They are able to identify familiar sounds, people and their surroundings from an early age. Sensory development, and the way in which a carer supports the five sensory aspects of sight, sound, touch, smell and taste, are key factors in baby care.

A baby's physical development, i.e. growth of the body in size (height, weight, head circumference) is measured and recorded on a centile chart (see Chapter 7, page 92) at regular intervals to monitor the rate of growth and physical development.

All babies have basic needs which should be met in order for them to grow and develop. The ages and stages of a baby's growth and the role of the carer are covered in Table 6.5 on pages 80–2, which is based on a model produced by Angela Dare and Margaret O'Donovan (1994).

BASIC NEEDS

The basic needs of the baby are evident towards the end of the birth process when the baby's head is being delivered. At this stage the midwife will begin to wipe away the mucus from the baby's mouth and nose. Within seconds of the birth, the baby will begin to breathe independently.

The needs at birth

Following birth, the baby is examined to determine whether there is an immediate medical need. The standard method adopted involves the use of the Apgar score. Five vital signs are checked:

- *heart rate* – is there a rapid heart rate? In babies this is above 100 beats per minute
- *breathing* – is the baby breathing? Is the breathing regular? Is the baby crying?
- *muscle tone* – is there movement? Can the baby move his body or different parts of his body?
- *reflex response* to stimulation – Is there a reflex action when the foot or nostril is stroked?
- *colour* – is the baby's colour healthy, giving the appearance of being fully oxygenated, i.e. oxygen has reached the different parts of the body? Sometimes the hands or feet are not fully oxygenated and may be slightly blue in appearance.

The checks are made 1 minute and 5 minutes after the birth. The signs are scored in points which are either 0, 1 or 2. The points are added up – the maximum score is 10 and most babies score between 9 and 10. If there are any concerns, then the Apgar score is continued at five minute intervals. A more detailed examination of the baby is carried out later.

As soon as possible after the birth, the baby is passed to the mother. The baby is then bathed and any distinguishing features which are present are noted (see the diagram opposite).

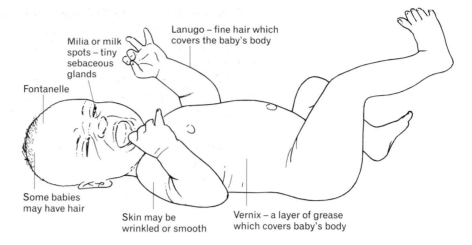

Milia or milk spots – tiny sebaceous glands

Lanugo – fine hair which covers the baby's body

Fontanelle

Some babies may have hair

Skin may be wrinkled or smooth

Vernix – a layer of grease which covers baby's body

The distinguishing marks of a new-born baby

Screening tests of the new-born baby

Soon after birth, and before the baby is allowed to go home, screening tests are carried out. When the baby is about six days old and has taken some milk feeds, a sample of blood is taken from the heel for the Guthrie test which detects:

- *phenylketonuria (PKU)* – an inherited disorder which is caused by the presence of excess phenylalanine in the blood. It results in damage to the nervous system and mental retardation. It can be successfully treated if it is noticed early

- *hypothyroidism* – a disorder of the thyroid gland which will affect future growth and development.

The baby's head circumference is measured, and her weight is recorded. The hips are examined for congenital dislocation of the hip, and a general examination is carried out to exclude other conditions or diseases.

Babies and diet

Breast and bottle feeding

The choice between bottle- and breast-feeding is an important one to make. It is often made during the antenatal period, i.e the period of time from conception to birth.

In some cases, the mother may decide to breast-feed but, following the birth of the baby, she may decide to opt for the bottle-feeding method instead. Whatever the decision, support should be given to the mother. Carers should not impose their own ideas with regard to feeding methods on the new mother. There may be a number of reasons why the mother may not be able to maintain the breast-feeding regime. For example, she may have cracked and painful nipples. The breast v. bottle debate is always a topic of conversation between new mothers. The main points are summarised in Table 6.1.

Whichever choice is made, a baby has nutritional and dietary needs which must be met if she is to grow and develop in the crucial first months of her life. All babies need a healthy and balanced diet (see Chapter 4, page 37).

Breast feeding	Bottle feeding
● Colostrum – a yellow syrupy mixture which is available during the first 10 days. It is high in protein. ● Breast milk, which is made in the breasts in the second to the fourth day. At first it mixes with colostrum which gives it a creamy appearance. ● It contains protein, fat, glucose, sugar and vitamin C. It is suited to the baby's nutritional needs. ● The baby can be fed immediately the need arises. ● Holding the baby against the breast and placing the nipple in the baby's mouth so that he can feed. ● Skin-to-skin closeness between the mother and baby promotes attachment and bonding. ● Careful washing of breasts before and after feeding. Some women rub lanolin on their nipples to prevent soreness. ● Winding after feeds.	● No artificial replacement for colostrum. ● Formula milk is necessary for all new-born and young babies and contains the nutritional requirements. ● Careful calculation of the feeds is essential. 75 ml of fully reconstituted feed for every 500 ml of a baby's weight in a 24-hour period, i.e. 2½ fluid ounces per pound every 24 hours. The total feed is then divided into the number of bottles. ● Holding the baby so that the teat is placed in the mouth for the baby to suck the milk from the bottle. The baby should never be left alone propped up on a pillow with a bottle. ● Sterilisation of bottles and feeding equipment using appropriate techniques. Hands should be washed before and after feeding and preparing bottles. ● Winding during and after feeds. The baby may suck in air as the bottle empties.

Table 6.1 The main features of breast and bottle feeding (adapted from Dare and O'Donovan, 1998)

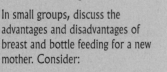

ACTIVITY

In small groups, discuss the advantages and disadvantages of breast and bottle feeding for a new mother. Consider:

● how much time each method takes – will the choice be different if the mother is returning to work?

● how involved will the father, or other members of the family, be in the feeding routine?

● how much is advertising involved in influencing parents in their choice in feeding?

Once a feeding routine has been set up, the baby will grow in size and develop and should put on weight. She will have increasingly longer periods awake but should also sleep for periods between feeds. However, when she is no longer satisfied after a milk feed, she may become restless, irritable and may begin to suck on her fists and fingers. This may be the time for the baby to be weaned.

Weaning

Weaning is the gradual introduction of a variety of solid foods into the baby's diet. To begin with, the baby may be offered a couple of teaspoons of baby rice mixed with milk. A teaspoon or a baby spoon is used and a very small amount of food is slipped into the baby's mouth.

The baby gradually gets used to the sensation of food in the mouth. It is often sensible to introduce one flavour at a time. At first the food will be bland and smooth, but as the baby acquires teeth and is able to chew more lumpy food may be given. As the weaning programme continues the baby develops likes and dislikes. A weaning plan is given in Table 6.2.

Weaning should be integrated into the family meal times. Offering the baby a spoon to hold so that she can learn to feed herself helps to develop her hand–eye co-ordination and fine motor skills.

At meal times, the baby should wear a bib, to catch any food or liquid which dribbles from her mouth.

Age/months	4 months	4½ months	5–6 months	6–7 months	7–8 months	9–12 months
On waking	Breast or bottle feed	Breast or bottle feed	Breast or bottle feed	Breast or bottle feed	Breast or bottle feed/cup	Breast or bottle feed/cup
Breakfast	1–2 teaspoons baby rice mixed with milk from feed or with water; breast or bottle feed	2 teaspoons baby rice mixed with milk from feed or with water; breast or bottle feed	Baby rice or cereal mixed with milk water or pureed banana; breast or bottle feed	Cereal mixed with milk from feed or water; fruit, toast fingers spread with unsalted butter	Cereal, fish or fruit; toast fingers; milk	Cereal and milk; fish, yogurt or fruit; toast and milk
Lunch	Breast or bottle feed	1–2 teaspoons puree of sieved vegetables and chicken, breast or bottle feed	Pureed or sieved meat or fish and vegetables, or proprietary food; followed by 2 teaspoons pureed fruit or prepared baby dessert; drink of cooled, boiled water or well-diluted juice (from cup)	Finely minced meat or mashed fish, with mashed vegetables; mashed banana or stewed fruit or milk pudding; drink of cooled boiled water or well-diluted juice in a cup	Mashed fish, minced meat or cheese with vegetables; milk pudding or stewed fruit; drink	Well-chopped meat, liver or fish or cheese with mashed vegetables; milk pudding or fruit fingers; drink
Tea	Breast or bottle feed	Breast or bottle feed	Pureed fruit or baby dessert; breast or bottle feed	Toast with cheese or savoury spread; breast or bottle feed	Bread and butter sandwiches with savoury spread or seedless jam; sponge finger or biscuit; milk drink	Fish, cheese or pasta; sandwiches; fruit; milk drink
Late evening	Breast or bottle feed	Breast or bottle feed	Breast or bottle feed, if necessary			

Table 6.2 A suggested weaning plan (Dare and O'Donovan, 1998)

The temperature of the food should be checked – it should not be too hot so that it burns the baby's mouth. Cold food, on the other hand, can be unappetising for a baby. The food should be thoroughly cooked – partially cooked and uncooked food may cause stomach upsets or food poisoning such as gastro-enteritis.

When weaning is introduced, a baby may experience some feeding problems. Table 6.3 explains how these can be managed.

Problem	Signs and symptoms	Management
Allergies and intolerances	Failure to thrive, diarrhoea and vomiting, infantile eczema/general rashes, wheezing	Liaise with medical advice/dietician Breast-feed if possible Use cow's milk replacement, for example, soya milk
Constipation	Small, hard, infrequent stools	Increase fluid intake Ensure feed not too concentrated No laxatives or sugar in feeds If weaned, increase fruit or vegetable intake Check to exclude underfeeding
Diarrhoea	Frequent, loose watery stools	Check hygiene of food preparation Give clear fluids and seek medical advice
Colic	Babies of (usually) less than 3 months cry and draw legs up appearing to have abdominal pain. Often showing distress at the same time of day – frequently early evening	Cause unknown Feed baby Check teat for size and flow, if bottle-fed Monitor feeding technique Reassure carer that pain is self-limiting Comfort baby with movement and cuddling Seek advice from health visitor
Overfeeding	Baby vomits/unsettled, passes large stools; sore buttocks, excessive weight gain	Seek clinic/health visitor advice Check re-constitution of feeds
Possetting	Baby frequently vomits small amounts, but gains weight and is happy	Condition self-limiting usually solved when baby is upright and walking Monitor weight
Underfeeding	Baby very hungry, wakes and cries; stools small and dark, poor weight gain; vomiting as a result of crying and air swallowing	Ensure feeds are correctly re-constituted If breast-feeding, check technique and mother's diet Increase frequency of feed, before quantities

Table 6.3 Problems associated with feeding (Dare and O'Donovan, 1998)

Warmth

A young baby has not developed the heat regulating system which is necessary for keeping her warm and to prevent her over-heating. She is not able to cope with cold temperatures and cannot shiver effectively.

Babies can be kept warm through regular feeding. This generates their body's metabolic rate, i.e. the different chemical reactions in the body which are necessary for it to function properly and to warm itself. The room temperature should be maintained at about 21 °C. The room should be warm when the baby is being washed, bathed or changed.

The baby's clothes should be appropriate to the environment and to the seasons. Babies require layers of clothes which can be taken off to prevent

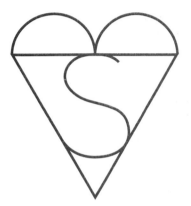

The British Standard kite mark

over-heating or added to when the baby feels cold. Warm blankets are needed at night and any drop in temperature should be taken into account and the room heating adjusted accordingly.

Security and protection

Babies should be kept safe at all times as they are particularly vulnerable to injury. They should never be left unsupervised when lying on an arm chair, for example, as they can move around and fall off.

Measures that can be taken to ensure their safety include:

- *straps and harnesses* – make sure that the baby is always strapped into a car seat, high chair or push chair. However, they should not be tied in too tightly

- *prams, carrycots, pushchairs, baths and cots* – all equipment should carry the British Standard kite mark to ensure that it is safe for use.

- *guards and gates* – need to be positioned over the stairs, in doorways, and to protect cooker plates. Window locks should also be fitted, and fires and heaters should be protected with guards

- *lockable cupboards* – to ensure that any harmful chemicals are not easily accessible

- *plug covers* – three-point electric sockets at low level should have a safety plug in place when they are not in use.

KEY POINT

Babies should never be left unsupervised as they have no instinct for danger or impending danger. This makes them particularly vulnerable to accidents.

Love and affection

The love and affection which exists between a young baby and his mother or primary care-giver is an important part of the **bonding** process – the close and developing relationship between a baby and the mother or primary care-giver.

Bonding may happen immediately following birth, when the baby and mother meet each other for the first time. In other cases, the process may gradually develop over a couple of months as a result of holding, cuddling, talking, kissing, smiling, tickling and other gestures which strengthen the relationship.

Bonding can be encouraged by:

- *eye contact* – the mother or primary care-giver and the baby can build rapport by looking into each other's eyes

- *skin contact* – skin contact between the mother or primary care-giver helps the baby to feel secure and get used to the familiar smell of his mother or care-giver

- *consistent and regular contact* – seeing the same face and learning to recognise it promotes a baby's sense of security

- *familiar routine* – maintaining the same routine every day, enjoying bath and feeding times with the same familiar people.

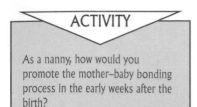

As a nanny, how would you promote the mother–baby bonding process in the early weeks after the birth?

The first relationship which a baby forms in the bonding process will be a contributing factor to other relationships which she will form when she grows older. Strong, affectionate and emotional bonds promote positive self-esteem and develop a sense of self-identity.

According to Erikson's life stages (see page 68), the baby is at *Stage 1 (0–1½ years): Basic trust versus mistrust.* The baby develops a trust in the familiarity of her surroundings. She is dependent on her main carers and needs to feel safe and secure. This trust has a fundamental part to play in a baby's emotional development. When babies are removed from their familiar surroundings, they can become anxious and distressed. They can begin to lose the sense of trust which they have built up (see Chapter 7, page 103).

KEY POINT

It is important to remember that individual babies will have different sleep patterns.

Rest and sleep

Sleep and rest are major factors in a baby's life since it is during these periods that the body grows and develops. Carers need to incorporate periods of rest into a baby's daily routine. These opportunities for rest enhance a baby's sleep patterns.

A baby will soon establish a familiar routine and sleep at set times during the day and night. Factors which enhance their sleep include making sure that they are warm, dry, comfortable and that they are adequately fed. Bedcovers should be loose and pillows should not be used as they are deemed to be unsafe.

As a baby grows older, her sleep pattern changes and she tends to sleep less during the day and to maintain her sleep period at night. A growing baby may sleep for approximately 12 hours a night. However, some babies require less sleep than others. This is particularly demanding for parents who may try many different tactics to encourage the baby to sleep.

There may be disruptions in a baby's night-time sleep patterns caused by:

- teething
- illness, for example, coughs, colds and difficulties with breathing
- changes in regular routine caused by visits, holidays, celebrations
- unfamiliar surroundings and noises.

Following a disruption in a baby's routine, she may find it difficult to return to the original routine. This should be encouraged as soon as possible.

CASE STUDY

Daisy

Janet and Richard have a young baby daughter called Daisy. At 6 months she suffered from a mild form of bronchitis (chest infection). Since then she has not slept well during the night, waking up every 45 minutes and crying for attention. Daisy is now 9 months old. Her parents are both exhausted.

1 What strategies would you introduce to encourage Daisy to sleep for longer periods at night?

2 How would you support Janet and Richard?

Exercise and fresh air

Alongside sleep, exercise is an important aspect in a baby's early months. Stimulating exercise will often encourage relaxation which enables the baby to rest and sleep more effectively.

Exercise can be promoted in the early weeks of life by encouraging the baby to stretch and move during bath time and nappy changing. Bath time is an ideal opportunity as the baby can move around unrestricted by clothing and nappies. The baby should be encouraged to kick its legs and move its arms.

Introducing the baby to fresh air and sunlight may be achieved by, for example, putting the baby outside in a safe place for a morning sleep or taking the baby to the park in the pram or pushchair. The baby should be well wrapped-up against the cold or well protected from the sun.

CARE ISSUES WITH BABIES

Promoting adequate care and ensuring that a baby is safe, secure and growing physically involves the management of various care issues.

Medical supervision

The medical supervision of a young baby commences before the baby is born. The care of the pregnant mother usually begins when the pregnancy is confirmed. This is generally carried out by the primary health care team – GP, health visitors and community midwives. The primary health care team is usually based at a health centre. The pregnant mother attends the health centre for:

- *regular monitoring* – to observe and record the health and well-being of the mother and foetus
- *screening* – taking blood tests and checking for any inherited disorders in the foetus.

When she attends hospital, the mother-to-be will be in the care of a consultant gynaecologist, hospital doctors, midwives and nurses. Following the birth, which may take place in hospital or at home, the mother and baby will be cared for once more by the primary health care team with each member having a different function (see Table 6.4).

GP/family doctor	Midwife	Health visitor
<ul><li>Care for the pregnant mother before, during and after the birth</li><li>Treat any illness of the mother and baby</li></ul>	<ul><li>Care for the pregnant mother</li><li>Conduct home birth if necessary</li><li>Visit and support mother and baby for up to 10 days following the birth</li></ul>	<ul><li>Visit new babies and their mothers regularly when the midwife has completed her visits</li><li>Offer support</li><li>Carry out regular child health surveillance at the clinic</li><li>Carry out screening and developmental tests</li><li>Responsible for health education</li></ul>

Table 6.4 The functions of the primary health care team

Health screening and surveillance

In the first year of a baby's life, she will be assessed at regular intervals at a child health clinic as part of **child health surveillance**. This involves growth and development tests, and screening tests.

Screening tests in the first year include:

- birth – screening tests of the new-born baby (see page 71)
- approx. 6 weeks – repeat examination of hips and testes
- approx. 6–8 months – vision checks
- approx. 7–8 months – hearing checks
- hips check before baby starts walking.

Immunisation

In addition to health surveillance, the baby will enter an **immunisation** programme. Immunisation is artificial protection against disease which is achieved by giving the baby either a very weakened dose of a specific disease, or by giving her some weakened toxins (poisons) which the disease produces.

Immunisations are given at 2, 3 and 4 months of age. Babies receive a course of immunisation of two doses each month so, for complete protection, the baby will have six injections. The primary course protects against:

- diphtheria, pertussis (whooping cough) and tetanus – the triple immunisation, known as DPT
- poliomyelitis (polio), given by mouth as drops on the tongue
- haemophilus influenzae type B (Hib).

By giving these mild doses over a period of three months the baby's body is gradually able to build up an ability to produce and reproduce antibodies to fight disease.

The Hib immunisation is different from the DPT injections because it stimulates the baby to produce antibodies against a bacteria that can cause several illnesses – the most serious being a form of meningitis. It is also effective against types of blood poisoning (septicaemia), infections in the bones and joints (osteomyelitis) and several forms of chest condition.

Protection against measles, mumps and rubella (MMR) is offered to babies between 12 and 15 months.

To ensure that the baby is able to produce these new antibodies safely, it is important that she is fit and well at the time of the injections. If the baby has any reaction to one of the immunisations, for example, running a fever or developing a swollen painful lump at the site of the injection, then the doctor may postpone further injections. In addition, if there is a history of fits in the baby's family, she would not given the pertussis injections (Dare and O'Donovan, 1998).

Developmental needs

As a baby grows, she develop various skills which become evident as she progresses through different stages. These stages of development all have necessary care needs. The baby's development has a number of aspects:

KEY POINT

A record of the immunisations a baby has received is given to the parent. This record is a useful way of keeping track of them.

- *Physical development/motor development* – physical growth of the body in size, i.e. height, weight, head circumference; these are measured and recorded on a centile chart (see Chapter 7, page 92). The baby develops gross and fine muscle controls which are known as motor skills. She learns to move her muscles and bones in a co-ordinated way. This produces mobility and is called locomotion (see the diagram below).

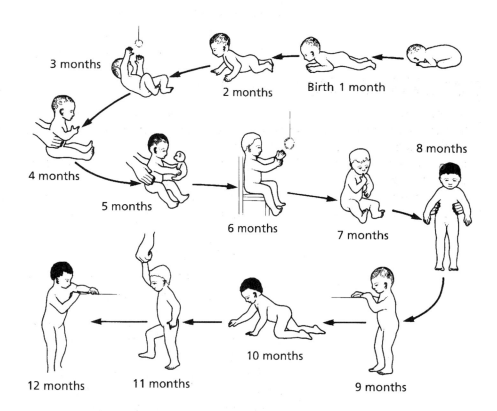

The development of locomotion (Dare and O'Donovan, 1998)

Babies have physical needs which include a healthy diet, hygiene, sufficient rest, sleep, space to move and a safe environment.

- *Intellectual and cognitive development* – development of the brain and reflex actions, recognition of people and objects, of memory and speech. Babies need to be exposed to sounds and language. Talking and singing to a baby stimulates learning.
- *Emotional development* – begins at birth with the bonding process. Holding and cuddling of the baby by familiar adults with positive reinforcement of smiles and eye contact support a baby's emotional needs.
- *Social development* – involves how a baby relates to others, her family and her living environment. Toys and play activities encourage and stimulate learning, and also encourage building rapport and relating to others.

- *Sensory development* – promoting development of the five senses:
  - *sight* – hanging objects such as mobiles, the baby watches the movement
  - *sound* – making noises, using rattles, clapping stimulates a baby's response
  - *smell* – encouraging a baby to use their noses and sense of smell; drawing their attention to smells, such as food and perfume
  - *taste* – introducing different tastes gradually such as ice cream, yoghurt, tomato sauce
  - *touch* – holding, stroking and feeling encourages closeness; experiencing different textures, soft, smooth and furry, developing a sense of touch
- *Cultural development* – a baby grows up in the culture of her family. The socialisation process and the family's child-rearing techniques will form part of her identity.

The role of the carer is crucial in meeting the individual needs of the baby. A model produced by Angela Dare and Margaret O'Donovan (1998) reviewed the stages of development and the carer's role, see Table 6.5.

Age	Development	Role of carer
Birth 4 weeks	• Motor development – will fix on faces and objects. Eyes follow bright moving objects. Lies supine with head to one side. Drops objects in hands, which are clenched. Reacts to loud sounds. • Language and social – throaty noises. Interested in faces. • Learning and emotional – reflex response, but becomes distressed by discomfort, for example cold. Enjoys feeding and cuddling. Great need to suck. Quietens when picked up.	Talk to baby, change tone, describe events. Baby enjoys mobiles and faces (visual range 20–25 cm). Hold, touch, fondle. Music, gentle movement. Use baby's name. Introduce to household noises and different rooms. Change position of cot. Use brightly coloured clothing and linen. Hold firmly, talk and sing to baby when feeding. Expect no set routine. Feed on demand.
8 weeks Posterior fontanelle closed	• Motor development – controlled movement beginning to replace reflex responses. Turns from side to back. Begins to lift head briefly from prone position. Shows eye co-ordination to lights and objects, squinting less obvious. 'Listens' to bell and 'stills'. • Language and social – begins to respond to adult's voice. Looks for sounds. Begins to coo and squeal with pleasure. Smiles in response to adult. Cries now begin to indicate type of distress • Learning and emotional – begins to recognise familiar face, more interested in own world. Enjoys sucking.	Use wind chimes and mobiles, the baby will watch the activity. Use bright colours in pictures placed in cot. Place in supporting infant chair to watch adult activity, or carry around. Use light rattles, let baby kick without nappies. Expose to different textures. Massage, and stroke limbs for example when bathing. • Talk and smile with baby, sing – allow time to respond • Talk to baby when feeding, hold close. • First immunisation. *continued*

Table 6.5 A summary of the stages of development (adapted from Dare and O'Donovan, 1998)

Table 6.5 continued

Age	Development	Role of carer
12 weeks Primitive reflexes now disappearing	• Motor development – baby rests on forearms when prone. Basic crawling movements, may get chest off surface. Shows preference for sleeping position. Holds objects in hands, brings to mouth, cannot release. Watches hands. Head control improved. • Social and language – generally sociable, smiles readily, babbles, coos. Stops when handled or sees known adult, turns head to follow. Enjoys playing when feeding. Stays awake longer. • Learning and emotional – recognises familiar faces and objects. Shows interest in own world and is aware of changes. Enjoys repetition of activities. Continues to enjoy sucking. Routine more settled, especially in sleeping.	• Encourage smiling, laughing. Place on changing mat on floor. Continue to widen sound stimulation. Take on outings well-protected. Develop rattle use, stimulate baby to attempt to reach for it and follow with eyes. • Immunisation programme continues.
16 weeks: stepping and rooting reflexes go 4–5 months birth weight redoubled	• Motor development – eyes focus on small objects. Holds head up when pulled to sitting. Beginning to reach for objects. Turns to familiar sounds. Sits with support. Rolls from back to side. Grasps with both hands. Everything taken to mouth • Social and language – laughs and chuckles socially. Recognises mother, seeks and enjoys attention. Begins to respond to 'no'. Enjoys being propped up. • Learning and emotional – enjoys attention, becomes bored when alone. Recognises bottle. More interested in mother, shows trust and security. Sleeps through the night, has defined nap time.	• Show baby mirror and encourage play. Give soft squeezy toys with different colours and textures. Water play in bath. Continue with rattles. Pat-a-cake, peek-a-boo games. Repeat sounds at varying levels. Introduce gentle 'rough and tumble'. Offer simple picture books, name items. • Safety – watch for toys that are too small, with loose fittings that might be swallowed. • Completion of primary triple and Hib immunisations
26 weeks (6 months): eye-to-eye contact. Palmar grasp replaces inferior pincer grasp at 6–7 months. Two lower central incisors appear	• Motor development – sits alone for a few seconds. Bounces and weight bears when held in the standing position. Transfers objects, and places in mouth with one hand. Enjoys playing with feet. Bags objects together, rolls over well. Possibly moving by rolling or squirming. • Social and language – recognises strangers. Squeals, laughs aloud. Double syllable babbling, starts to say Ma, Da. Talks in 'own' language in conversation with adults.	• Provide toys to bang, stack and nest (round ones easier). Saucepans, spoons, 'safe' household equipment. Continue with peek-a-boo, bye-bye, pat-a-cake. Provide opportunities for developing large movement, space, firm furniture. Provide music and movement, simple repetitive rhymes. Give pouring and squeezy toys to play with in bath. Continue with picture books. Extend outings to include animals, for example feeding the ducks. Imitate animal sounds. Let baby copy you – building bricks, etc. Allow time, not hurrying. Offer cup and extra spoon at mealtimes. Strap into high chair, give finger foods but allow to 'play' with own food.

continued

Table 6.5 continued

Age	Development	Role of carer
26 weeks (6 months) *continued*	• Learning and emotional – looks for objects that are out of sight. Curious, handles and looks at objects closely. Knows where sounds originate. Pulls toy with a string. Drops and picks up toys. Continues to mouth and bite. Shows fear of strangers and is upset when mother leaves. Continues to explore food. Enjoys sitting in high chair.	• Safety – look at wider environment, for example plugs, electrical equipment baby can reach with increasing mobility
40 weeks (10 months) Four upper incisors – 9 months	• Motor development – sits unaided, can regain balance. Manipulates objects with hands. Unwraps objects. Pulls to stand in cot, creeps. Uses finger and thumb to hold objects. • Social and language – claps hands when asked. Knows own name, copies facial gestures and sounds, smiles at self in mirror. Aware of environment, will play alone for considerable periods. Indicates likes and dislikes at meal and bedtimes. • Learning and emotional – begins to imitate. More interested in books. Wishes to be more independent in dressing, feeding, etc. Enjoys achievement.	• Allow baby to make choices in play material. Offer balls, dolls, pull and push toys, sand and water trays (well-supervised), building blocks, music. Teach names of body parts. Continue to extend experiences including types of foods, textures and tastes. Encourage baby to return affection.
12 months 10–14 months: Anterior fontanelle closing. Birth weight triples. Two lower lateral incisors, and four first molars appear by 14 months	• Motor development – cruises around furniture, begins to start alone, able to manage stairs. Begins to walk unaided. Turns pages in book. Builds tower of two blocks. Puts ball in box. May use spoon. Can release objects voluntarily. Shows preferred hand. Attempts to throw. Regular bowel movements. • Social and language – uses jargon, points to indicate wishes. Enjoys give and take games. Enjoys music, being noticed, having achievement clapped – will repeat for actions. • Learning and emotional – shows fear, anger, affection, jealousy, anxiety and sympathy. Determined in approach to play, increased concentration and attention. Some idea of space, time and effects of own actions.	• Motion toys – provide carrying and moving toys. Continue with sand, water and music. Continue to extend all activities and language. Allow child-directed play in a safe environment. Encourage self-feeding, use of cup and spoon. Manage unacceptable behaviour with firm quiet 'no'. Distract if possible. Give and encourage return of affection.

Care routines

Routines are an integral part of caring for babies. Baby-care routines include:

- hygiene routines (see below)
- feeding routines (see below)
- play routines – introducing the baby to a colourful environment, attaching mobiles which move, rattles, cuddly teddy bears. These should be introduced after a rest period during the day
- rest and sleep routines – including a regular rest period, and having regular bed times and waking times.

Hygiene routines

The purpose of hygiene routines is to keep the baby clean and comfortable.

- *Nappy changing* – a baby's nappy should be changed at regular times during the day. It is important that the baby's bottom is washed and dried thoroughly before a clean nappy is put on. Have all the equipment ready before you start. Follow this procedure:
  1. Wash your hands and put on a pair of protective gloves.
  2. Lay the baby on a changing mat.
  3. Remove the soiled nappy, lifting the baby's legs by the ankles. Dispose of the nappy in a nappy bag or bin provided for the purpose.
  4. Wipe the baby's bottom with wipes or moistened cotton wool.
  5. Wipe and gently dry the genital area.
  6. Put on a clean nappy. Dress baby.
  7. Make baby comfortable in a safe place, such as a cot.
  8. Clean all surfaces, put equipment away, remove and dispose of gloves and wash your hands.

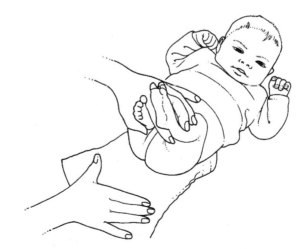

The baby is placed on a clean nappy

- *Topping and tailing* – washing the baby's face and hands and changing the nappy.

- *Bathing* – giving the baby a full bath using either a baby bath for younger babies or the big bath for the older baby. Have all the equipment ready and check the temperature of the bath water before you start (see the diagram below). Follow this procedure:
  1. Lay the baby on a flat, safe surface, undress her and remove the nappy.
  2. Wrap the baby in a towel so the arms are tucked in.
  3. Wash her face with moist cotton wool.
  4. Hold the baby over the bath and wash her hair.
  5. Remove the towel.
  6. Lower the baby into the bath, holding her securely.
  7. Wash the baby with your spare hand.
  8. Lift the baby out of the bath, dry her, put on a clean nappy and dress her.
  9. Make the baby comfortable in a safe place, while you clean up.

KEY POINT

Babies are vulnerable to infection so, before and after a routine, the carer should always wash their hands.

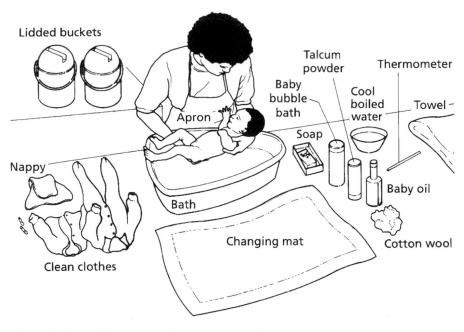

Equipment for bathtime (Dare and O'Donovan, 1998)

Feeding routines

These involve preparing bottle feeds and, later, meals once the baby is being weaned. Hygiene is an important consideration in feeding routines. The diagram opposite shows how to prepare a bottle feed.

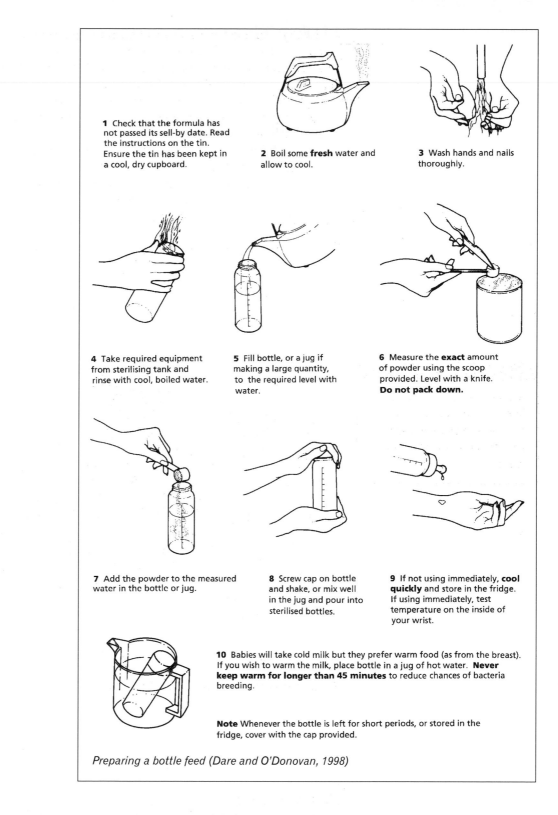

1 Check that the formula has not passed its sell-by date. Read the instructions on the tin. Ensure the tin has been kept in a cool, dry cupboard.

2 Boil some **fresh** water and allow to cool.

3 Wash hands and nails thoroughly.

4 Take required equipment from sterilising tank and rinse with cool, boiled water.

5 Fill bottle, or a jug if making a large quantity, to the required level with water.

6 Measure the **exact** amount of powder using the scoop provided. Level with a knife. **Do not pack down.**

7 Add the powder to the measured water in the bottle or jug.

8 Screw cap on bottle and shake, or mix well in the jug and pour into sterilised bottles.

9 If not using immediately, **cool quickly** and store in the fridge. If using immediately, test temperature on the inside of your wrist.

10 Babies will take cold milk but they prefer warm food (as from the breast). If you wish to warm the milk, place bottle in a jug of hot water. **Never keep warm for longer than 45 minutes** to reduce chances of bacteria breeding.

Note Whenever the bottle is left for short periods, or stored in the fridge, cover with the cap provided.

Preparing a bottle feed (Dare and O'Donovan, 1998)

LIFE EVENTS

In a baby's life there will be predictable and unpredictable events. How the baby and her mother, father or primary care-giver cope with these changes is important.

Predictable events

Predictable events are nevertheless ones which affect babies as they grow and develop. Coping with predictable events is part of daily living. Some examples are given in Table 6.6.

Event	Method of coping
Meeting the birth family members, friends and professional carers, such as health visitors and doctors	Regular contact with baby so faces are familiar
Visiting places, shopping, attending clinic, going on holiday	Ensuring the baby can observe what is going on; talking to the baby
Mother may return to work and another carer will look after the baby	Allowing a period of time for the baby to become familiar with their new carer and surroundings, if a day nursery or child-minder's home is being used

Table 6.6 Examples of predictable events during infancy and methods of coping

Unpredictable events

In a new baby's life there may be unpredictable events which occur. It is when unpredictable events occur that coping is more difficult. Coping strategies are necessary to support the baby and her carers. Some examples are given in Table 6.7.

Event	Method of coping
Premature birth	Baby is admitted to special care unit; parents will visit and give support
Birth injury	Baby is admitted into medical care; the short-term and long-term effects are discussed and decided
Birth mother is seriously ill and separated from baby	A substitute person, for example, the father or another family member, will care for baby and build up an attachment
Baby born in adverse circumstances and abandoned	Baby is cared for by medical staff and social services. The baby is sent to foster parents where relationships can be built up

Table 6.7 Examples of unpredictable events during infancy and methods of coping

Coping strategies are an important aspect in a carer's role. Part of the strategy may be to support a baby's family through the following stages when they are:

1   in denial; disbelief at the event, 'it's not true'
2   beginning to identify the problem or situation

3 feeling the effects of the situation, long term and short term
4 confronting the feelings, however negative they are
5 needing information, i.e. the opportunity to learn from others
6 making decisions for the future
7 looking for resolution and a way to move on in the situation.

In different circumstances and situations in a young baby's life, it is clear that loving carers and a safe and stimulating environment are key factors in supporting a baby's development and growth.

SPECIAL AND ADDITIONAL NEEDS

A baby may have a **special need** at any time prior to the birth and following the birth. A special need is a condition which may affect a baby's health and well-being on a short-term or long-term basis, i.e. it can be a temporary or permanent condition.

A special need can affect a baby's physical, emotional, intellectual, cognitive, sensory and social well-being. Examples of special needs include the following.

- *Inherited diseases and disorders* – diseases and disorders which are passed on to children from their parents. They are always present at birth but they are not always easily identifiable. Hereditary disorders include phenylketonuria (PKU). Other factors may be chromosomal inheritance, such as Down's syndrome, or sex-linked inheritance, such as haemophilia (which only affects boys).

- *Birth injuries* – which occur during the delivery of the baby and may result in permanent or temporary damage to the bones, muscles, nerves and skin of the baby. Bones can fracture, nerves can be stretched and damaged, particularly the nerves which supply the neck.

- *Sensory impairments* – which affect sight, hearing, smell, taste and touch, for example, loss of hearing, visual disturbance or numbness in a limb or limbs.

- *Failure to thrive* – a disorder which occurs when a baby does not appear to grow at the expected rate. Reasons for this condition include a possible feeding disorder, if the baby is not sucking properly. The baby may be allergic to milk, or may have difficulty in absorbing food. Other factors may be that the baby is prone to infection or receives little or no stimulation in the home environment.

- *Persistent crying* – when a baby may be crying for long periods and it is difficult for the carer to calm or soothe the baby. This may be due to teething, infection or allergy, but sometimes there is no obvious reason.

- *Infection or illness in the early months of life* – the baby may develop a cough leading to bronchitis or contract meningitis and hospital care may be necessary.

- *Abuse* – the baby is subject to different forms of abuse (see Chapter 7, page 108).

KEY POINT
Babies with special needs have the same basic needs for love, protection and security as other babies. They develop their individual identities as others do.

SOURCES OF SUPPORT

Support agencies may be statutory or voluntary organisations which provide a service for individuals, families and groups in society. There are a number of different types of support network and agency, offering a range of services, which include:

- *sharing information* – supplying leaflets, research statistics, videos and advice sessions
- *counselling* – telephone help lines, immediate crisis support and one-to-one support
- *group support* – meeting others with similar experiences
- *professional and specialist support* – through hospital specialist or groups such as the National Childbirth Trust.

Informal support networks

These consist of different networks involving families, friends and neighbourhood groups.

Formal support agencies

These are professional contacts who offer support to the young baby and her family. They include health visitors and GPs. Most agencies offer specialised support, for example, with parenting and breast-feeding. For example:

Association for Postnatal Illness, 7 Gowan Avenue, London SW6 6RH

Child Growth Foundation, 2 Mayfield Avenue, Chiswick, London W41 PW

National Childbirth Trust, Alexandra House, Oldham Terrace, Acton, London W3 6NH

National Society for Phenylketonuria (UK) Ltd, 7 Southfield Close, Willen, Milton Keynes, MK15 9LL

Twins and Multiple Birth Association, PO Box 30, Little Sutton, South Wirral, L66 1TH

```
     ┌────────────────────┐
     ╲    KEY TERMS    ╱
      ╲                ╱
```

KEY TERMS

You need to know the meaning of the following words and phrases. Go back through the chapter to make sure that you understand them.

birth injuries
bonding
child health surveillance
failure to thrive
immunisation
inherited disease
phenylketonuria (PKU)
sensory impairments
special need
weaning

Self-help groups

These offer assistance to individuals and their families who are experiencing difficulties in relationships or who may be suffering from isolation and loneliness. For example:

Association for Breast Feeding Mothers, 26 Holmshaw Close, London SE26 4TH

Families Need Fathers, 134 Curtain Road, London EC2 3AR

KIDS, 80 Waynflete Square, London W10 6UD

Mother's Union, Mary Sumner House, 24 Tufton Street, London SW1P 3RB

Meet a Mum Association (MAMA), 58 Malden Avenue, South Norwood, London SE25 6HS

National Council for One Parent Families, 255 Kentish Town Road, London NW5 2LX

7 *Caring for children*

PREVIEW

Caring for children requires a knowledge of how children develop and how their different needs are met in a variety of care settings. This chapter will enable you to develop your understanding of:

- Growth and development
- Basic needs
- Care issues
- Life events
- Special and additional needs
- Sources of support.

Caring for children and meeting their individual needs is a worthwhile occupation. Young childen have a great capacity to be interested in the world around them. They are keen to learn how things work and to understand the different aspects of the society in which they live.

As carers and care workers, it is interesting to observe young children as they learn and play together. Observation of children is a way of assessing a child's individual growth and developmental needs.

GROWTH AND DEVELOPMENT

Childhood is a period of rapid physical growth and development. Carers and child-care workers find that a basic understanding of the different stages of a child's development helps them to work more effectively with the children in their care. This knowledge helps in the assessment of a child's individual needs. Table 7.1 outlines child development in the following age groups:

- 1–2 years – the toddling years
- 3–5 years – the pre-school years
- 5–10 years – school age.

Age	Physical development	Intellectual/cognitive development	Emotional development	Social development
1–2 years Toddler stage	• Can pull themselves up to a standing position • Walks around holding on to furniture before they have the courage to let go and walk • Walks very fast and tends to fall over • Can climb stairs and come down backwards • Holds a spoon • Can feed themselves using fingers • Lifts cup to mouth	• Uses up to 50 words and can put together simple sentences • Refers to themselves by name • Can build a tower of up to seven cubes • Uses both hands but hand preference is beginning to be recognised • Enjoys looking at books and pointing to objects • Enjoys conversation games such as song and rhyme	• Is curious about the world around them • Tends to be very dependent on adults • Will play alongside another child but not with them • Finds it difficult to share with others • Wants adult approval and praise	• Makes effort to join in with adults and others when they sing to him • Swings between being dependent to being independent and wilful • Can be unco-operative and difficult • Can be loving and responsive
3–5 years Pre school stage	• Runs and climbs • Uses a tricycle and can cycle round corners • Kicks a large ball • Walks upstairs using alternative feet • Sits with feet crossed in front of them	• Can use up to 3,000 words over this period • Talks fluently and asks many questions • Can state their full name and knows their age • Can copy a circle and a cross • Uses scissors and pencil	• Develops confidence and is less likely to have tantrums • Displays of frustration are reduced as language and vocabulary increase • Enjoys praise for achievement	• Can play with others and take turns. • Can play alone for periods in order to develop a new skill • Enjoys imaginative play • Shows concern for other children who are upset or have hurt themselves
5 years + School age	• Uses large apparatus to climb, swings on ropes. • Skips using a rope • Dances in time with music • Can balance on poles • Enjoys PE in school	• Uses a pencil with competence • Begins to learn to read stories • Can draw a circle • Concentrates on different tasks • Introduced to the different topics included in the school curriculum • Completes key stages 1 and 2 of the National Curriculum	• Enjoys praise for achievements • Able to concentrate for periods and work in isolation • As they grow older can begin to be self-critical and this can affect confidence and self-esteem • Finds failure hard to accept	• Relates with other children • Makes friends and may have one particular friend • Can work on projects with other children, can show initiative but still expects intervention and support from an adult

Table 7.1 Stages of development in the child

A child's growth is monitored and recorded on a growth chart or centile chart (see page 92). By doing this, potential problems can be identified at an early stage and be treated accordingly.

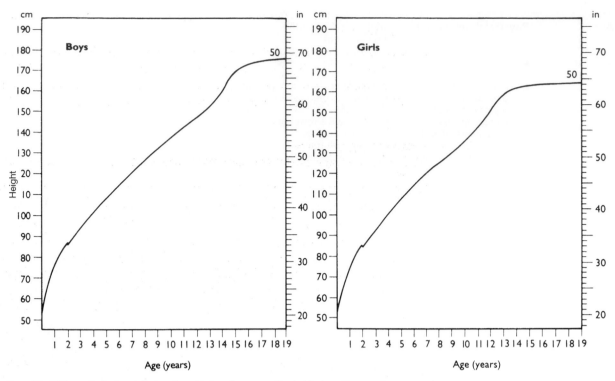

Note: The 50th centile for length is given from birth to 2 years, and for height from 2 years of age onwards.

Examples of centile charts

BASIC NEEDS

The basic needs of children cover the same issues that have been identified in previous chapters. It is important to remember that the needs of children are universal and that they should be met, regardless of a child's cultural and ethnic origin, social class and family background.

Balanced, healthy diet

A growing child needs a balanced and healthy diet in order to maintain physical growth and development. The components which contribute to a healthy diet are discussed in Chapter 4 (page 37).

There are a number of factors which affect a child and their diet, including:

- *a child's personal likes and dislikes* – children develop likes and dislikes for certain food, for example, they may not like green vegetables, but have a preference for burgers and chips. There is nothing wrong with such preferences, but carers especially need to ensure that the child eats some fruit and vegetables, which contain essential vitamins and minerals

- *the family income and financial status* – the family may not be able to afford fresh food and vegetables and this can be restrictive in supporting a healthy diet

- *peer group pressure and advertising pressure* – children notice that their friends like certain foods and they want to have the same. The latest advertisement on television offering a new breakfast cereal with a toy or other gift often provides an incentive to eat a particular brand of food.

CASE STUDY

Jenny

Jenny is 7 years old and loves ballet and tap dancing. She enjoys jumping up and down to the beat of the music and attending classes at the local dance school. Last week, two other girls started giggling at Jenny as she was dancing. Although Jenny appeared her usual self, her mother has now noticed that she is 'off her food'. She refuses to finish a meal and says she is not hungry. Her mother has been worried about her, and has arranged a check-up with the doctor. Although the medical check found no problems, Jenny is still not eating.

1 What do you think has happened in this situation?

2 How would you support Jenny?

3 How would you reassure Jenny's mother?

4 How would you encourage Jenny to eat a meal?

5 What are the long-term effects on Jenny's health if she does not start eating properly?

Personal hygiene and toileting

From an early age children should be learning about their bodies and how to manage their own toileting and hygiene needs. Learning to wash their hands before and after meals is important, as well as after going to the toilet. There are different strategies which may be employed to help children with their own care routines, as follows:

- *Toilet training* Introducing a potty at an appropriate time, supervising and giving praise for results.
- *Daily washing routines at home* Washing is introduced as part of a child's day and is carried out at certain times during the day. In the morning a child will get up, wash their face and hands and clean their teeth.

At first they may need the help and supervision of an adult until they can manage themselves. In the evening, they may have a bath or shower before going to bed. Other families may shower in the morning. Whatever routine is adopted, children should be taught to respect their bodies and keep themselves clean.

- *Equipment within easy reach* A child should be able to reach the wash basin to wash their hands and should have access to hand-drying equipment. Standing at the toilet can be difficult for a small boy so a step should be provided. Soap, flannel, toothbrush and toothpaste should be placed within easy reach. In school and at other care provisions, the same guidelines should apply. Enabling a child to learn to wash and toilet themselves is an important step to independence.

- *Adjustable clothing* A child should wear clothes which are easy to pull down or unfasten for toileting purposes. Elaborate belts and buckles can complicate the act of going to the toilet and children may wet themselves in the process of getting undressed. Learning to dress and undress themselves allows children to become independent.

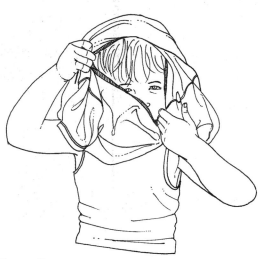

Look at me, I can do it myself

- *Access to toilets and wash basins in school* As part of the settling in process to any care provision, the child should be shown where the toilets are. It can be particularly upsetting if the child gets lost trying to find it. Wherever possible a named and responsible worker should show the child around when they first arrive. As a safety precaution, a child should never be taken to the toilet by a person who is not a worker, teacher or carer.

It can be seen, therefore, that a growing child needs support with their different physical needs. As they mature, they learn to manage these tasks for themselves.

Physical exercise

Physical activities promote a child's physical growth. As soon as physical skills such as walking are achieved, they should be practised so that the child develops onto the next stage, such as running, hopping, skipping and jumping.

Physical skills should be encouraged at every opportunity. This prepares a child for life and helps their body mechanisms to co-ordinate physical movements. The different skills which are developed are:

Physical exercise is an excellent way in which to promote bodily development because it:

- strengthens and stretches muscles which improves muscle tone and encourages co-ordination

- stimulates the appetite, helps the food digestion process and reduces constipation

- helps a child's breathing by encouraging the lungs to expand, which in turn supports the healthy functioning of the heart

- creates a feeling of well-being and builds up self-esteem.

- *gross motor skills* – large body movements which enable the child to develop confident, physically active and well co-ordinated body movements. Opportunities should be offered to meet these needs, such as walking, running, manoeuvring a tricycle or bicycle, climbing, swimming and gymnastics. All these activities promote stretching and improve the mobility of the body's joints, bones and muscles. Providing equipment for indoor and outdoor play helps to promote these skills

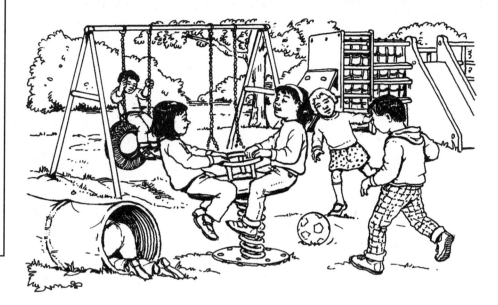

Physical play is fun!

- *fine motor skills* – small body movements such as hand–eye co-ordination in which the child can hold and examine a small object by moving it into their line of vision. These fine movements are encouraged by, for example, teaching a child to use a knife and fork, dress themselves, do up buttons, hold pens and pencils, use scissors, catch a ball or hit a ball with a bat

- *spatial awareness* – supporting a child to use the space around them helps the development of fine and gross motor skills. For instance, a child learns to slow down when approaching a large object in her path. A child who is painting starts by covering the whole page in one colour, then as she develops a sense of space starts to paint objects in a variety of colours using different brushes.

Security and protection

Looking after children and keeping them safe from accidents is an important concern for carers. Accidents are a major problem for children between the ages of 1 and 14. A significant number of accidents occur at home.

ACTIVITY

Describe how you would make a large room in a community centre safe for a group of 6-year-old children to carry out physical play activities.

The physical environment in which children play, live and learn should be safe. This can be addressed by:

- *providing a safe indoor environment* – all household equipment which is potentially dangerous should be locked or provided with guards, such as fire guards, cooker guards and stair gates. As children get older, it should not be taken for granted that they can manage. Careful instructions should be given, explaining why there is a need for safety. This includes supervision during cooking activities

- *providing safety outdoors* – children enjoy being outdoors, but this should be carefully monitored and supervised. Play areas should be free of dangerous items such as broken bottles and rubbish. A growing concern for parents is the way in which children's play areas may be unsafe due to the presence of strangers. Children should also be taught about 'stranger danger' and also how to be safe on the roads

- *ensuring that workplace safety policies and procedures are met within the various care provisions* – organisations should be working within the statutory requirements laid down in their organisation's health and safety policy. This includes the provision of adequate first aid equipment and the availability of a qualified first aider to carry out first aid procedures. Other requirements include locking up dangerous substances and maintaining the prescribed adult : child ratios.

Rest and sleep

As children grow older, they still need adequate rest and sleep. Bedtimes may be later for the older child but most still require at least 10 hours of sleep a night.

Older children often do not have established rest times; they may attend after-school clubs or take part in extra curricular activities, such as learning a musical instrument. These can make a child tired by the end of a school week.

ACTIVITY

How would you ensure that the following children have adequate rest and sleep:
a) a girl aged 4
b) a boy aged 7
c) a girl aged 10.

Intellectual stimulation and play

Children have an in-built sense of curiosity. They are interested in learning about how things work and discovering the world around them.

To support a child's intellectual and cognitive development, it is important to stimulate their curiosity, as this supports their learning. The first stages of learning are often incorporated into play. It is in these early stages of play that a child learns to use their reasoning and problem-solving skills.

Play occupies a child in activities which promote development and learning in a pleasurable and satisfying way. Through play, children attain skills and knowledge which support their personal development. As children grow and develop, they move through different stages of play, from simple activities, such as moulding dough, to more complicated activities, such as setting up a game of monopoly with a group of friends.

Play stimulates growth in various developmental aspects (Beaver, Brewster and Keene, 1997):

- *physically* – it encourages movement and control in gross and fine motor skills
- *intellectually and cognitively* – it leads to the development of thinking, including conceptual thought, problem-solving, creativity, imagination, memory and concentration
- *linguistically* – it stimulates the development of verbal and non-verbal communication skills
- *emotionally* – it can provide the opportunity to experience and express a range of emotions and to learn how to control them
- *socially* – it enables children to develop the skills they need for interaction with others. This includes learning to share, co-operate, take turns and make friends
- *morally* – it helps children to learn the existence of rules, and how to conform to them. Through play, they can gain a sense of what is right or wrong and can develop a conscience.

Play has many functions and purposes. Individual children play in different ways – some quietly, others noisily and actively. Despite these apparent differences, children generally adopt distinctive styles of play according to their age, as follows.

- **Solitary play** (0–2 years) – children will play alone, although they like to have a parent or carer in the background.
- **Parallel play** (2–3 years) – children enjoy playing independently alongside each other.
- **Associative play** (3 years+) – the child begins to play with others in small groups. At this stage, children learn to share and interact with others, but they will still sometimes revert to solitary and parallel play.
- **Co-operative play** (3 years+) – children play and learn together giving each other roles and responsibilities within the group. They may set up and play games using rules.

ACTIVITY

A youth leader has asked you to set up a play session for a group of five children aged 7. Describe:

a) the activity you would choose, stating your aims and objectives

b) the resources and materials you would need

c) how you would set it up

d) the skills you would hope to develop

e) how you would evaluate the activity

f) what the health and safety implications of the activity are.

There are many types of play, all of which develop particular skills in the child. Ideally, the child should have the opportunity to participate in all these different types of play throughout childhood. Examples include:

- *creative play* – involving different materials, such as paint, water, sand and collage
- *constructive play* – using bricks and Meccano
- *make-believe play* – involving role play and imaginative play. Children imitate adult actions and enjoy dressing up and using role play, for example, playing hospitals
- *problem-solving play* – using games and puzzles
- *hobbies* – computer club, football, chess, dance and music.

Many children under the age of 5 attend pre-school groups or nurseries where activities are set up to promote learning. From the age of 5 years, or during the rising 5 year in most areas, children begin a more formal approach to learning and attend school.

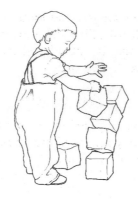

Solitary play

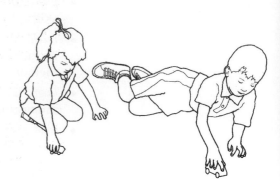

Parallel play

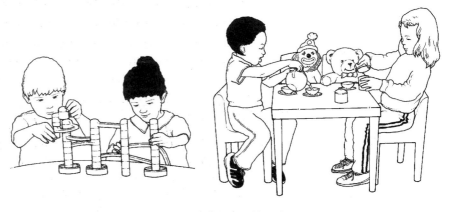

Associative play

Co-operative play

In school children receive instruction in reading and writing (literacy) and in maths and number work (numeracy). Children's learning is guided by Government standards which are set out in the **National Curriculum** – the curriculum which must be taught to all children of statutory school age (i.e. 5–16 years) in the UK.

The National Curriculum is divided into four stages:

- Key Stage 1 – 5–7 years
- Key Stage 2 – 7–11 years
- Key Stage 3 – 12–14 years
- Key Stage 4 – 14–16 years.

The Curriculum is made up of five core subjects:

- English, Mathematics and Science, which are the subject of Standard Assessment Tests (SATs) at the end of each Key Stage, and
- Religious Education (RE) and Information and Communications Technology (ICT), which are not tested by SATs.

In addition, there are six foundation subjects at primary level: History, Geography, Art, Music, Physical Education (PE) and Design and Technology. A foreign language is introduced as a seventh foundation subject at secondary level at the age of 11.

Love and emotional security

The need for love and affection is important to the growing child. The knowledge that they are loved unconditionally by their primary care-giver is vital. Such unconditional love is a result of the positive bonding process which was discussed in Chapter 6 (page 75).

As well as meeting a child's emotional needs, a carer should understand that children have certain statutory rights which include (Beaver *et al.*, 1999):

- having their needs met and safeguarded
- being protected from neglect, abuse and exploitation
- being brought up in their family of birth wherever possible
- being considered as an individual, to be listened to, and to have their wishes and feelings taken into account when any decisions are made concerning their welfare.

This is supported by the United Nations Convention, 'The Rights of the Child' (1991).

The United Nations Convention: The Rights of the Child

This Convention sets out a number of statements which support the rights of children and young people. It states that children have three main rights which should be considered whenever a decision is being made about them, or any action is taken which affects them. These are:

- *non-discrimination* – all the rights in the convention apply to all children equally whatever their race, sex, religion, language, disability, opinion or family background (Article 2)
- *best interests* – when adults or organisations make decisions which affect children, they must always think first about what would be best for the child (Article 3)
- *the child's views* – children, too, have the right to say what they think about anything which affects them. What they say must be listened to carefully. When courts or other official bodies are making decisions which affect children, they must take note of what the children want (Children's Rights Development Unit, 1993).

In addition to the acknowledgement of their individual rights, a child needs to know that they are loved and valued. The carer and care worker have important roles to play in supporting a child's emotional security. They can do this by:

- *encouraging a child to express their feelings* – when a child is feeling excited about an event or incident in their lives, the carer should encourage them to share this feeling. Equally, when a child is unhappy, frustrated and withdrawn, the carer should take the child quietly to one side and talk to them gently in a reassuring manner. A gentle and sensitive approach will support the child in sharing his upsets

- *providing a child with a secure environment* – children enjoy following a routine. They like to see the same faces, familiar tasks and activities in a familiar setting. This makes them feel secure. When these surroundings are to change, carers should always prepare a child in advance whenever possible. Changes should be introduced gradually; for example, when a child transfers from nursery to school, the carer should talk to the child about the change, take her for a visit in advance to meet other children and the new teacher

- *building a child's self-esteem, confidence and sense of achievement* – praising a child for their achievements. There is no task too small that cannot be praised

- *helping a child to develop methods of coping with anxieties and difficult experiences* – talking to a child about the different events and changes which have happened and allowing feelings to be shared is important. A child may often take her lead from familiar adults in times of crisis.

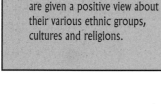

ACTIVITY

In small groups discuss and decide:

a) how you would teach a child about different cultures

b) how you would ensure that a class of 25 children aged 9 years are given a positive view about their various ethnic groups, cultures and religions.

Development of identity

Showing a child affection and love helps them to develop their self-identity or self-image. This means that they develop a view of who they are. Building a positive self-image is most important in the life of a child.

A positive self-esteem may often be reliant on response from others. Primary care-givers and adults working with children should value a child and their contribution and give them praise for their efforts and achievements.

Children tend to see themselves in relation to their surrounding environment and therefore it is important that the child has a positive view of their social, cultural and religious background. This can be achieved through visual displays, books, photographs, drawings, artwork and activities such as cooking. The influence of culture on a child's developing identity is an important one.

The development of a personal identity is reviewed in Erikson's theories with regard to childhood (see the table on page 68). It touches on three areas:

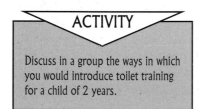

ACTIVITY

Discuss in a group the ways in which you would introduce toilet training for a child of 2 years.

- *Stage 2 (1½–3 years): Self-control versus shame and doubt* During this stage, the children are developing more muscle control. They are becoming more independent and need to learn a certain amount of self-control. They may become frustrated if they do not get their own way. Some children have tantrums at this stage. This is often the time when a baby tries to become a child but still has the needs of a baby. Potty and toilet training is introduced at this stage. It should be managed by the parent or care-giver in a positive, flexible way. A child will have accidents until they have established a routine and have become toilet-trained.

- *Stage 3 (3–7 years): Initiative versus guilt* Children are now becoming more confident in how to use their bodies, and they are able to take initiative and promote ideas. This is an important stage for a child, because it is now that they can become particularly sensitive to their environment. For instance, a child's understanding and physical development can be affected by deprivation. A child needs space to play, people to communi-

KEY POINT

At this stage, language and culture play an important part. If a child does not have a clear understanding of the predominant spoken language in an area, they can feel self-conscious, with implications of 'feeling different'.

cate with and opportunities to learn from new experiences. In a home where a child has little or no stimulation to learn and grow, the way they relate to themselves and to others will be damaged.

- *Stage 4 (6–15 years): Industry versus inferiority* In this stage the word 'industry' refers to children working, problem-solving and being concerned with how things are made. They are developing new skills and competence, i.e. the ability to carry out a variety of tasks and activities which stimulate their learning. This is an important time for children who consistently need to be given encouragement and positive reinforcement about their new skills and achievements. It is important this encouragement is given by teachers and other adults. As a child is supported in their achievements, they begin to feel valued as individuals.

CASE STUDY

Supporting a child starting school

Hussein is 5 years old. He has just moved to England from Bangladesh. His first language is Syletti, a language spoken in Bangladesh. It is his first day at school and his mother had visited the school on previous occasions in order to help Hussein settle into his class. When his mother leaves, however, Hussein becomes very distressed. What would you do to support Hussein?

1 What would be your first consideration?

2 How would you communicate with Hussein?

3 What are the immediate issues?

4 What strategies would you introduce to develop Hussein's learning?

CARE ISSUES

Behaviour management

An important issue in child care is the management of a child's **behaviour**. Behaviour relates to a child's conduct, to acceptable and unacceptable ways of carrying out actions and speaking to others. Children's behaviour should be challenged within the boundaries of what is expected. This is called discipline, or behaviour management.

Behaviour can be acquired through learning from others in different ways such as:

- *awareness of the expectation of others* – such as parents, family members, friends, teachers and other carers
- *imitating others* – children often watch how others behave and may copy that behaviour
- *identifying with others* – children value the friendship of their peers and this may influence their actions
- *reinforcement* – children learn by reward or by retribution. For example, a child will learn to behave if they are given praise and encouragement in

what they are doing. This is called positive reinforcement. If they are constantly being told to be quiet or to go away then they will not have a clear idea of what is expected. This is called negative reinforcement.

According to Beaver, Brewster and Keene (1997):

'normal behaviour is the behaviour which is to be expected at a particular age. A framework for children's behaviour provides the agreed approach to how children should be encouraged to behave within a childcare setting.'

It involves setting goals and boundaries based on values. These define what is considered to be acceptable conduct. Normal behaviour will be dependent on:

- the characteristics of the individual child
- the child's family, social and cultural environment and the expectations placed on the child within that environment
- whether the child has any individual special needs, for example, a physical impairment or learning difficulty.

Setting goals and boundaries is about creating a relevant framework relating to the acceptable behaviour which is to be encouraged.

- The goals of behaviour should cover all aspects of conduct within the care setting. This includes social, physical and verbal behaviour, for example, how a child behaves in the setting, how they behave towards themselves, other children, parents, other carers and teachers. It is important that this framework is appropriate to the ages of the children.
- Boundaries are the limits set and considered as defining acceptable behaviour. Children should know that if they cross this boundary they will be disciplined or sanctioned.

How children's behaviour is managed relates closely to their emotional developmental needs. How these needs are met is often dependent on the relationship which a child has with their parents and primary care-givers.

Separation anxiety

When a child becomes separated from their parents for a variety of different reasons, such as hospitalisation, the child may suffer from the effects of separation. John Bowlby (1951), a child psychologist, believed that:

'the infant and young child should experience a warm, intimate, and continuous relationship with his mother (or permanent mother-substitute) in which both find satisfaction and enjoyment.'

Bowlby carried out research with James and Joyce Robertson in which they identified that there were stages experienced by a baby or young child when they are separated from their parents. They suggested that a child between 6 months and 4 years of age is particularly vulnerable to the effects of separation. The stages of separation are as follows.

1 *Protest* The child is grief-stricken, calling constantly for the parent(s).
2 *Despair* The child sinks into apparent depression, becoming quiet, apathetic and withdrawn, mourning for the lost parent(s). The child may adopt self-comforting behaviours, such as thumb-sucking, and may regress developmentally, for example in potty training, play activities or language.
3 *Denial* The child no longer appears depressed and shows interest in the immediate surroundings. The child may now repress all feelings for the parent(s). If the child has a prolonged hospital stay, he may settle into the routine and way of life. The child will turn away from familiar adults, such as parents.

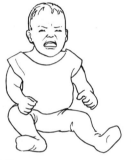

1 Protest

The young child is angry at being separated from his mother, father or primary care-giver.

2 Despair

The young child is not able to understand that his mother, father or primary care-giver will return.

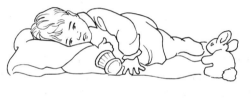

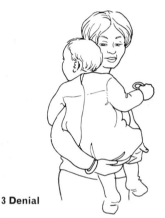

3 Denial

The young child denies the existence of the mother, father or primary care-giver.

The stages of separation

Children suffering from separation need support, care and sensitivity. In some cases, a carer may work specifically with the child to give them a sense of security and familiarity. If possible, careful explanation should be given to the child to help them understand what is happening. Positive reminders, a comforter or transitional objects will help to remind the child of the love and affection of their parents and that they will be returning.

Social contact and relationships

Positive relationships which a child builds with a carer enable him to make and maintain social relationships with others. Most children enjoy meeting other children. Observing groups of children in a school playground talking, playing and communicating, provides many insights into their behaviour.

As a child grows older, peer friendships, for example, those of fellow pupils, are very important. They want to be like their friends, imitate their behaviour, have the same lunch box and watch the same television programmes. This may sometimes lead to friction at home as families have varying values. For instance, some children may go to bed earlier than others.

The role of the carer and care worker can support a child in their relationships with others by developing the child's:

- *language skills* – from an early age introducing conversation, pictures, books, song and rhyme and music; talking to a child and listening to what they are saying and using activities to stimulate language, for example, on a bus ride, showing the child the different views from the bus window. Language is a satisfying way in which children can quickly and easily relate to each other

- *reasoning and problem-solving skills* – giving a child age-appropriate tasks to promote their problem-solving and reasoning and involving other children in these tasks. However, carers should always match the task to the child's ability

- *creativity and imagination* – providing a range of creative play activities to interest and stimulate a child's learning, for example, providing a child with dressing-up clothes and encouraging a group of children in imaginative play

- *observation and discovery skills* – encouraging the child to look at the world in which they live, for example, the changing seasons. Taking children for walks in the park, planting a garden, sowing seeds and watching them grow.

Young children find it difficult to listen to each other. The role of the adult is important here – they can encourage children to stop what they are saying, to look at the other person and to listen.

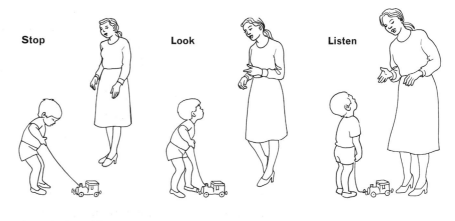

Stop, look and listen

The use of books and stories increases and develops communication skills both through speaking and gesture. Music is another way in which children can communicate noise, fun and enjoyment.

Children learn very quickly in a positive environment. They learn by watching and imitating their adult carers and teachers as well as their families and friends. At school. the teacher often becomes the 'expert' and often a mother is told 'Miss Lewis says...' even if the mother holds a different view. The feeling of independence and friendship-building closely identifies how inter-related emotional and social development occurs as children grow.

Self-help skills

Helping a child to communicate and relate to others is an important focus of their daily lives. They want to fit in and to achieve. Part of this process is ensuring that the child learns a number of **self-help skills**. These are skills which are necessary to carry out different tasks and activities to maintain daily living and independence (see also activities of daily living, Chapter 4, page 36, and living skills, Chapter 5, page 53).

In order to help a child to be independent, there are a number of skills which should be taught to a child before they go to school. These include:

- recognising their own name – show them their names on each item of their school clothes

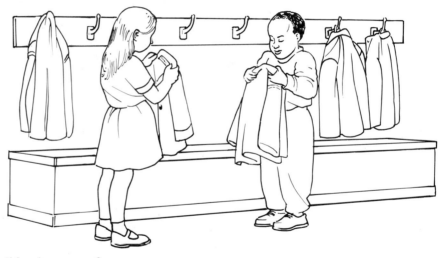

Is this mine or yours?

- ensuring that they can use the toilet, undress and dress as appropriate
- learning to identify the right order of clothes when they get dressed – lay out clothes in order when they get undressed. Before and after PE the child who has learned to organise their dressing and undressing will feel more confident. Learning which shoe goes on which foot is also helpful
- being able to hold a pencil and to know how to use a pair of scissors. If the child is left-handed, their needs will differ from the right-handed child; it is also important that left-handed scissors are supplied.

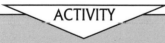

ACTIVITY

Look at the pictures on page 106. Discuss and decide the approximate appropriate age for each one.

These are simple steps which can make it easier for children during an important transition in their lives. These skills should be taught in a supportive and methodical way with lots of positive praise and encouragement.

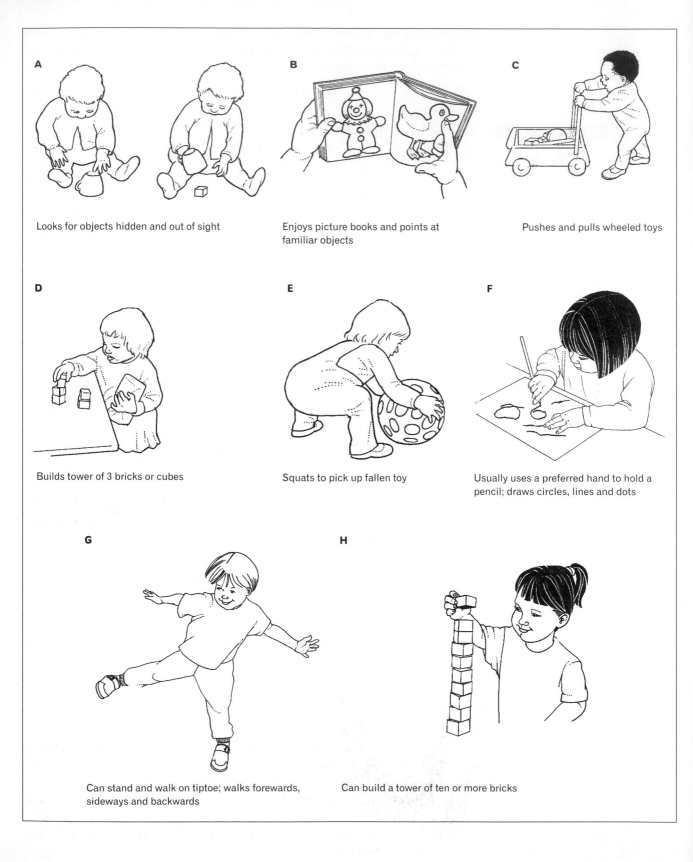

A Looks for objects hidden and out of sight

B Enjoys picture books and points at familiar objects

C Pushes and pulls wheeled toys

D Builds tower of 3 bricks or cubes

E Squats to pick up fallen toy

F Usually uses a preferred hand to hold a pencil; draws circles, lines and dots

G Can stand and walk on tiptoe; walks forewards, sideways and backwards

H Can build a tower of ten or more bricks

Children need adults to help and support them in their daily tasks and activities. This enhances a child's personal development. The carer can help and support a child by:

- *developing a child's awareness of the needs of others* – encouraging a child to watch and listen to other children, encouraging children to take turns in games and to share toys and equipment
- *enabling a child to relate to their peers and to make friends* – helping children to make friends with others by asking their names, sharing their favourite book, toy or television programme. Encouraging children to find shared interests is also important
- *enabling the child to interact and communicate with adults* – children will often imitate adults. They will watch and observe how a carer relates to their parents, or vice versa. Carers should provide positive role models in order for children to learn.

LIFE EVENTS

Predictable events

Examples of predictable events which occur in a child's life are given in Table 7.2.

Event	Method of coping
Birth of a sibling	Keep the child informed and include them in the different tasks and activities in preparation for the birth. Make sure they feel included once the baby has been born.
Starting school	Make sure that the child visits the school in advance, and meets the teacher and other children. Talk to the child about school and help them prepare their school bag and clothes.

Table 7.2 Predictable events in a child's life and methods of coping

Unpredictable events

We will look in detail at two unpredictable events which may occur in a child's life:

- being admitted to hospital
- **abuse**.

The child in hospital

The results of the research of Bowlby and the Robertsons (see page 102) led to the Platt Report (1959), *The Welfare of Children in Hospital*, which made recommendations with regard to children in hospital.

Many children are admitted to hospital each year. This can be an anxious and stressful time for them and for their parents. Parents may react in different ways to their child's hospitalisation. If the child is very ill, the parents' reactions may include:

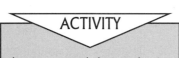

- *disbelief* – 'this can't be happening', especially if the illness is sudden
- *guilt* – 'Why is he ill? Was it something I did?'
- *anger* – parents may display feelings of anger towards the medical team and nurses caring for their child
- *fear and anxiety* – relating to a child's illness and to the different investigations and treatment which are being performed
- *frustration* – when parents feel that their sick child is not getting any better and that they are being given insufficient information about the child's illness
- *depression* – which can occur during the child's stay in hospital. This does not disappear when the child is discharged home. During a child's hospitalisation parents may become mentally and physically exhausted.

Following discharge, a child may have difficulty in adjusting to the home routine. The child may be confused, fearful of being hurt, and may revert to baby-like behaviour, which is known as regression. They may be worried and anxious about missing school.

A number of factors affect the child while in hospital, but it is equally important to remember that they will also affect the child's behaviour after they return home. The role of the carer is important in this situation.

Child abuse

Child abuse is the deliberate ill-treatment of a child. It can take many forms:

- *physical abuse* – non-accidental injury, i.e. physical harm to the child's body, shown by marks such as bruising in places not likely to have occurred accidentally, scratches, bites or cigarette burns
- *sexual abuse* – involving a child in a sexual actvity with an adult. A child might act out sexual activities in role play with a teddy or doll. There may be soreness, bleeding or itchiness around the child's genital area
- *neglect* – a child is not given basic care and may be unhappy or withdrawn or aggressive. He or she may have health problems and/or problems at school, such as truancy. The child may look unkempt, with signs of poor care, for example, failure to thrive or severe nappy rash
- *emotional abuse* – the child is subject to name calling, negativity and is likely to appear withdrawn and nervous. Personality changes may be evident and the child may have difficulty forming relationships.

Carers and care workers sometimes find it difficult to recognise abuse or to accept that it is happening. However, the behaviour of a child who changes in personality from being outgoing and happy to being withdrawn and silent is a cause for concern.

At all times it is important to mention concerns to a manager and never act alone. There are professional codes of conduct for dealing with cases of suspected abuse. If abuse is suspected, the social services department is informed.

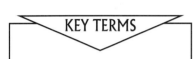

KEY TERMS

You need to know the meaning of the following words. Go back through the chapter to make sure that you understand each one of them.

associative play
behaviour
child abuse
constructive play
co-operative play
creative play
fine motor skills
gross motor skills
make-believe play
National Curriculum
parallel play
peer group
self-help skills
solitary play

SOURCES OF SUPPORT

The different types of support were discussed in Chapter 6, page 88. There are a number of agencies available to support young children, and to support the families of young children.

The professional support from health visitors, GPs and teachers is an invaluable means whereby most parents can feel that the individual growth and development needs of their children are being met.

Examples of support organisations for parents and young children include:

Barnados, Tanners Lane, Barkingside, Ilford IG6 1QG
Child Accident Prevention Trust, 4th Floor, Clerks Court, 18–20 Farringdon Lane, London EC1R 3AU
ChildLine, Freepost 1111, London N1 0BR
Contact a Family, 170 Tottenham Court Road, London W1P 0HA
Kidscape, 82 Brook Street, London W1Y 1YG
National Children's Bureau, 8 Wakley Street, London EC1V 9QE
National Council for One Parent Families, 225 Kentish Town Road, London NW5 2LX
Parentline UK, Endway, The Endway, Hadleigh, Essex SS7 2AN

CHAPTER 8

Caring for adolescents and teenagers

PREVIEW

Adolescence is viewed as the gateway to adulthood. During the teenage years many changes occur in the body, mind and emotions of a young person. This chapter will enable you to develop your understanding of:

- Growth and development
- Basic needs
- Care issues
- Life events
- Special and additional needs
- Sources of support.

The teenage years are often viewed by historians of childhood as 'the state of [young people] preparing themselves for adulthood by experimenting, studying, resisting, or playing' [Modell and Goodman, 1990].

Adolescence is a period of transition which begins with puberty and ends with the onset of adulthood. The period of adolescence is roughly between the ages of 10 and 18, but the time of onset varies from one individual to another.

Puberty is the period during which secondary sexual characteristics develop and the reproductive organs become functional, enabling an individual to reproduce. In girls, puberty usually starts between the ages of 10 and 13, while in boys it usually starts a little later, between 12 and 14 years. The onset of puberty is determined by many factors, including heredity and diet.

GROWTH AND DEVELOPMENT

Growth and development during adolescence is rapid because of the biological changes which are taking place in the body. In some cultures this is viewed as a cause for celebration and marked with a special ceremony. For example, Jews celebrate the Bar Mitzvah as the Jewish adolescent boy is welcomed into the synagogue and is given adult male status.

Physical development

At birth, **primary sexual characteristics** are present in all babies. The physical changes which occur in the body during puberty, due to an increase in the production of hormones, lead to the development of **secondary sexual characteristics** – the primary reproductive organs grow and mature. The changes are summaried in Table 8.1.

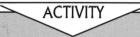

ACTIVITY

Design a poster for a group of boys and girls aged 10 years which explains the physical changes which occur in adolescence.

Primary sexual characteristics (present at birth)		Secondary sexual characteristics (develop during puberty)
Boys	Testes Penis Scrotum Prostate gland Seminal vesicles	Growth of axillary hair, chest and pubic hair Growth of penis, scrotal sac and testes Ability to ejaculate 'Breaking' of the voice
Girls	Ovaries Fallopian tubes Uterus Vagina	Breasts grow and develop Pubic and axillary hair appears Widening of the pelvis Menstruation begins

Table 8.1 Primary and secondary sexual characteristics

During adolescence the physical changes may have psychological effects. With their rapid physical growth outpacing their emotional development, some adolescents may feel clumsy and self-conscious about how they look. There is an increased production of oil and sweat producing glands which may lead to the development of skin conditions such as pimples and acne.

Puberty and adolescence is also a time of increasing sexual awareness. A girl will start her periods and a boy may experience ejaculation. Both these events are an indication that the adolescent boy and girl are sexually mature and that they are now able to reproduce.

The duration of these changes varies from person to person. It is important to remember that those physical changes which determine sexual maturity are different to the development of emotional maturity. Although the body is growing at a rapid rate, emotional development is not progressing at the same pace – few adolescent boys and girls are emotionally ready for the responsibility of parenthood, for example. Serious relationships in the adolescent years can be difficult simply because of the slower rate of emotional growth and development.

The constant changes in the physical state and the emotional demands of adolescence can lead to mood swings. See *Emotional development* (page 112) and *Emotional needs* (page 118).

KEY POINTS

Research has shown that during adolescence:

- girls mature earlier than boys. For example, the average onset of the height spurt for girls is around 10.5 years, whereas for boys it is about two years later

- the biological processes of puberty are spread over a long time. For example, breast growth takes place over a four-year time span

- the age for the onset of adolescence varies. For example, in a research sample on girls of 12–18 years, the mean age for the onset of menstruation was 13 years but the range ran from 10–16.5 years (Barnes, 1998).

Emotional development and the search for identity

Adolescence is a period when young people develop their own sense of identity or their sense of self. They are very aware of themselves – for instance, how they look, how they feel and how they relate to their peers is extremely important. In fact, this self-interest may lead to self-absorption, when the only issues which are important relate to their daily lives and interests. Therefore, adolescents find it difficult to understand that others may have different viewpoints. This can often make them inflexible in their approach to adults. For this reason, they may relate more easily to those peers, or group of friends, who share similar views to themselves.

This self-interest in adolescence is an indication of the need to develop individual identity. An aspect of this will often involve adolescents asking themselves the question 'Who am I ?' as they try to make sense of the adult world that they are moving towards.

Emotional development in adolescence and throughout the teenage years is about the maturation or 'growing up' which takes place within the different boundaries set by others. These boundaries, which are generally set by parents, teachers, other adults and friends, include time-keeping, study and homework times, balancing a social life with their education. Working within these boundaries may produce a sense of frustration. The teenager may feel that the boundaries set are too restrictive. The adults involved should encourage the teenager to talk about these frustrations. However, in some cases, talking may lead to further disagreement and debate.

On the other hand, as part of this process, some teenagers may hold strong views about the direction that they are taking and resent and find fault with authority figures. As children they may have worshipped their parents, but during the adolescent years they realise these people are far from perfect and often say so. Some parents can find this upsetting, while others view it as a necessary stage in the cognitive and emotional development of their teenage son or daughter.

As adolescents stretch their reasoning ability, they can become argumentative. Adults can play a useful role, if they involve adolescents in conversation and discussion without the emphasis on the adolescent's emotions but rather on their communication and cognitive approach to the discussion.

The relevant stage described by Erikson (1968) is *Stage 5 (13–21 years): Identity versus role confusion* in which the individual has to develop a consistent sense of who they are. Erikson postulates that rapid growth disturbs the previous trust which the individual had in his (or her) body and the understanding gained of the body functions that were enjoyed in childhood. The individual has to grow into this new body.

The unsuccessful resolution of conflict in its early stages can have lasting consequences by leaving unsettled issues to interfere with ongoing psycho-social development. Positive resolution of conflict can support an individual in the way that he or she is able to adjust to the demands of adolescence while retaining a sense of personal identity (Clarke, Sachs and Ford, 1995). Furthermore, changes relate closely to the young person's sense of identity. During this process they readily take on aspects learned in childhood but reject others. This can lead to conflict with others such as parents. Conflicts with parents tend to centre around homework, clothes, hairstyle, late nights out and relationships with peers.

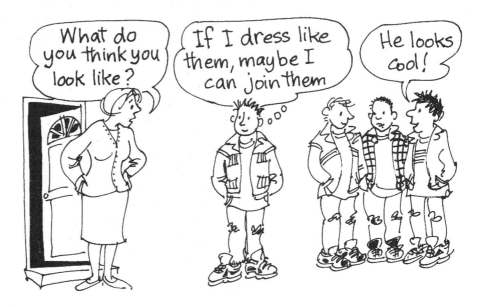

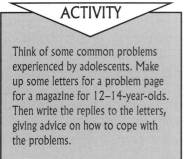
During adolescence a teenager may fall in love for the first time, spending every waking minute thinking about the object of their affection. During this period of infatuation, the adolescent may see only the good points until the time when the other person appears less than perfect. Then feelings can change drastically and may result in irritation, dislike, and disbelief that they could have ever been attracted to such a person in the first place.

Social development and social relationships

Building relationships is an important feature during the teenage years and adolescents may experience changes in how they relate to different individuals with whom they have contact. Social relationships include those with parents and friends, and personal relationships.

Parents

Adolescents are going through several changes themselves so changes in other people around them may provide even more stress. They find it difficult to understand that relationships involve work and commitment if they are to succeed. During the teenage years some youngsters have problems in relating to their parents. The cause may often be that young people want to assert themselves, become independent and part of this may be to reject the values of their parents.

CASE STUDY

Miranda

Miranda is 15 years old and lives with her parents in a large detached house in an affluent residential area. Her parents would like her to go to university like the sons and daughters of their friends. Miranda finds academic study very difficult and finds it hard to live up to her parents' expectations. She wants to train as a hairdresser and works at a local hairdressers on Saturdays. She feels constantly that her parents are not taking her feelings into account and she regularly argues with them. Miranda plans to leave home as soon as she is 16 years old. How would you support this family?

1 What advice would you give to Miranda's parents?

2 How would you support Miranda?

3 What care services would you involve in this situation?

Whilst in some ways adolescents find decision-making difficult, they can also be very decisive about their friends and leisure pursuits.

Parents may also suffer from fear for their child's safety, that their children will repeat the mistakes they themselves made and they may try, fruitlessly, to stop their children finding out the hard way; or some parents may react by feeling jealous of their child's freedom and lack of responsibilities, and long to be young again themselves.

Personal relationships

Adolescents form relationships with others which may or may not develop into a sexual relationship. It is important to discuss the responsibilities of forming such a relationship – the feelings and needs of two people are involved and should be considered. The boy may be more easily sexually aroused than the girl. She may view intercourse as much more than just part of the relationship and may find it difficult to understand the boy's demands for 'going all the way'. It is important that such a couple should learn to consider each other's feelings and attitudes in a relationship. If they work together to overcome their difficulties, their friendship can strengthen and develop. They will begin to realise that this is an important aspect of a loving and stable relationship which has positive benefits for them both.

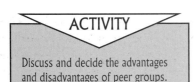

ACTIVITY

Discuss and decide the advantages and disadvantages of peer groups.

Peers

Friends of the same age and interests are very influential in the lives of adolescents – nobody wants to be different. Peer groups of adolescents may look for a common identity, which may be based on a pop culture or on a current interest. Friends are often made with people of similar tastes and outlook. But, as they grow older and reach their twenties, young people become less dependent on a group identity because they have formed their own independent opinions, views and beliefs.

Building positive social relationships is extremely important to teenagers. It closely relates to their intellectual and cognitive development.

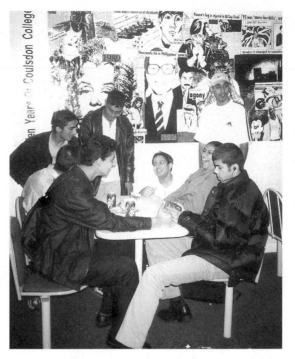

Being part of the peer group is important for the adolescent's self-esteem

Intellectual and cognitive development

Intellectual and cognitive development in adolescence has implications for social and emotional development. Strategies used by educators, teachers and others may have a profound effect on the way in which an adolescent may learn. Therefore the relationships with teachers, parents and others may either enhance or detract from the learning process.

Education and learning

In secondary school, adolescents are directed on how to learn and what to learn. As they grow older, they need to make choices about subjects to study and their possible future career.

Teenagers are encouraged to make decisions and to take control of their own learning. Secondary school is often the centre of the organising experience in most teenagers' lives. They gain new information, develop new skills and mature existing skills which should widen their views and attitudes to life.

Cognitive development

Adolescents need to develop reasoning and problem-solving skills. They should be able to read and write with confidence. They should be encouraged to conduct one-to-one conversations and join in peer group discussion. Their numeracy skills continue to develop. Other subjects are introduced into their curriculum such as foreign languages. They should be able to apply what they are learning to every-day situations.

Many adolescents enjoy using a computer for school work, playing computer games, finding information using a CD-ROM or scanning the Internet.

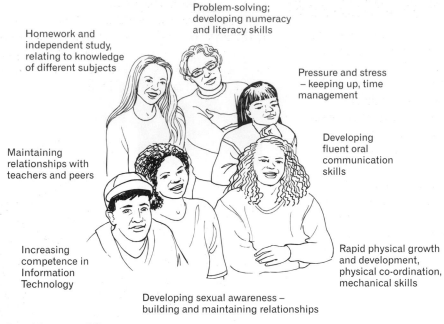

Problem-solving; developing numeracy and literacy skills

Homework and independent study, relating to knowledge of different subjects

Pressure and stress – keeping up, time management

Maintaining relationships with teachers and peers

Developing fluent oral communication skills

Increasing competence in Information Technology

Rapid physical growth and development, physical co-ordination, mechanical skills

Developing sexual awareness – building and maintaining relationships

Acquiring new skills

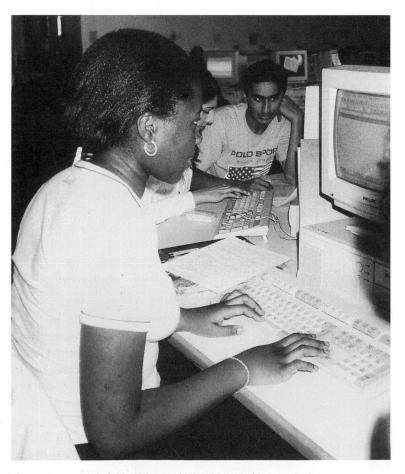

Computers are useful learning tools in all areas of the curriculum

Thinking about the future

It is during adolescence that individuals are encouraged to think about their future and their adult life. Different ideas will be developed and encouraged, or discouraged by parents, teachers and peers. Some teenagers may find it hard to make decisions, so having to make choices about careers or further education can be very difficult.

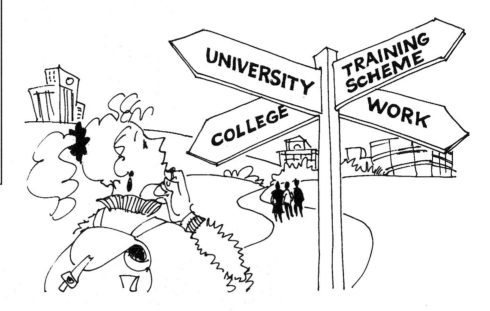

Making decisions about the future

BASIC NEEDS

Adolescents grow and develop in many different ways already discussed in this chapter. At each stage, adolescents have basic needs.

Physical needs

Adolescents have different physical needs. A teenager needs to have:

- *an understanding of the physical changes in the body* during adolescence – girls should know about their periods and how to use sanitary protection. Discussions about period pains and pre-menstrual tension (involving mood swings) will help a girl to understand her body and how it works. Equally boys should be able to discuss their physical changes, such as hair growth, shaving, wet dreams (ejaculation of semen whilst asleep) and erections of their penis

- *sex education* – information with regard to sexual relationships should be shared and the dangers of an unwanted pregnancy carefully explained. The Health Education Authority provides videos, leaflets and other forms of advice with regard to sexual relationships and contraception

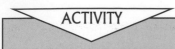

- *diet* – a balanced and healthy diet should be encouraged as this supports the adolescent's rapid physical development. Eating a low-fat diet with plenty of fruit and vegetables can help a spotty skin. Healthy diets are discussed in in Chapter 4, (page 37).

Positive social relationships

It is important for teenagers to identify with friends and peers. Peer groups can:

- have positive effects on teenagers' growth and development. For example, being in a group who do not 'do drugs'
- support each other's interests and help each other through difficulties and problems. They like to love and to be loved in return.

Equally they need to develop positive relationships with adults – they enjoy unpatronising and supportive behaviour from adults. A school or college tutor can play an important role in the life of a teenager who is finding communication with parents difficult. It can help them through a negative phase. Some schools and colleges offer a counselling service for pupils and students to talk about their problems.

Emotional needs

All adolescents have emotional needs. These relate to:

- *personal space and time* – adolescents like having personal space and time to themselves. They frequently enjoy being alone in their rooms, listening to music, for example
- *a sense of achievement* – all adolescents want to achieve, no matter what defences they put up. The role of a teacher or lecturer in building positive self-esteem and a sense of achievement is important. Some adolescents appear angry, defiant, uncommunicative and resistant to learning. Others are enthusiastic, hardworking and anxious to achieve.

Often a low sense of self, or negative self-esteem, can create a negative learning pattern. The adolescent, parent and teacher may set up a negative cycle in which the parents and teachers become more angry and frustrated and the adolescent becomes more defiant. In such cases, strategies should be designed to develop the learning process. A number of questions should be raised, such as 'What are the expectations of the adults concerned?' and 'What are the realities for the young person involved?' In most cases, a resolution can be found but this is not always the case.

It is interesting to note that the resolution to these learning difficulties may come in later life. Adults may choose to return to learning and to re-enter the education system as mature students.

KEY POINT

Supporting young people to develop a sense of achievement and positive self-esteem is a demanding task for those involved in working with them. Being encouraging and willing to listen is important. Furthermore, setting boundaries for appropriate behaviour is essential.

CASE STUDY
Roberta

Roberta is 16 years old. She left school with mostly grades D and E in her GCSEs. She managed to secure a place at her local college. During the first term, she is constantly late for lessons and does not contribute to discussion with the other students regarding course matters. However, during break time, she is seen as being very lively and communicative with her peers. One morning she arrives late in tears and in a quiet moment tells her course tutor that she has quarrelled with her parents and that she wants to leave home.

1 What are the issues involved here?

2 How would you support Roberta?

3 What advice would you give to the course tutor?

4 What specialist support should be available to Roberta?

CARE ISSUES

Carers and care workers working with young people require a variety of skills in order to identify their needs and give support. For instance, adolescence can be a most difficult period for parents, who frequently feel at a loss when their 16-year-old daughter slams the door and stomps upstairs yet again.

Adolescents can be moody. Such moods range from being very happy and talkative and, at other times, quiet and withdrawn. Exploring different strategies of support is a valuable requirement in maintaining communication and contact with the adolescent. There are times when an adolescent may need support with physical problems such as acne, hygiene and weight disorders.

Assistance with physical problems

Skin problems

Skin problems such as spots, or 'zits' (acne), and blackheads are the result of hormonal changes during adolescence. Such problems are regarded with despair simply because of their effect on the teenager's appearance.

Adolescents need to be reassured that the spots will disappear in time, but often that is no comfort while the spots are evident. Acne may affect the face, back and chest. In severe cases, it can lead to pitting and scarring on the skin. Treatment can involve using a variety of creams, anti-bacterial washes, and ointments which are available from chemists.

Those affected with acne should be encouraged to eat a healthy balanced diet rich in vitamin C. Cutting down on high-fat foods, such as chips, is also helpful. Squeezing and touching spots may lead to infection. Obviously this can make matters worse especially if the face is affected.

ACTIVITY

Visit the chemist, or the medicines area of the local supermarket, and research the different types of medication which are available for the treatment of acne. Which would you recommend to a group of adolescents?

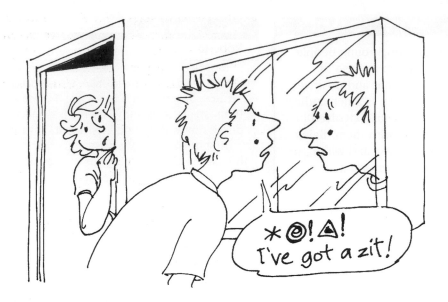

Weight problems

Adolescents may become preoccupied with their weight, their looks and what they and others are wearing. This can be a source of much anxiety, especially for girls.

Fashion models with perfect bodies wearing the 'proper gear' appear in advertisements in magazines and on television. This can promote a false image to an adolescent girl who instantly begins to feel fat and ugly, or skinny and unattractive. The effect may be that she becomes obsessed with slimming and in some severe cases may stop eating altogether. This may result in an **eating disorder** (see page 123).

In other circumstances, a young person may feel that they do not fit in with others. They will isolate themselves from their peers and become preoccupied with eating large amounts of food, leading to obesity. In this situation, the more self-conscious the young person becomes, the more they eat. Providing information about interesting and nutritious diets may be a start. However, if the problem is far deeper, specialist counselling and advice may be necessary.

Hygiene

During adolescence, the hormonal changes in the body prepare the individual for adulthood. There is a greater need for the individual to keep themselves clean. Adolescents have passed the stage where they need to be reminded to wash – although there may always be some who are happy not to bother! Carers should be aware that, for those who want to look and smell nice, there are some facts that need to be understood.

- Girls should know that the vagina has natural secretions which keep everything clean, so there is no need to wash inside it. However, once secretions reach the air, they are broken down by bacteria, and may smell unless the area is washed regularly with mild soap and water.

- Boys need to keep themselves clean because they may transmit thrush and bacterial infections to their partners during sexual intercourse. It is particularly important that uncircumcised boys learn to keep the area beneath the foreskin of the penis washed and clean. Lack of hygiene in this area has been identified as a contributory cause of cervical cancer in women.

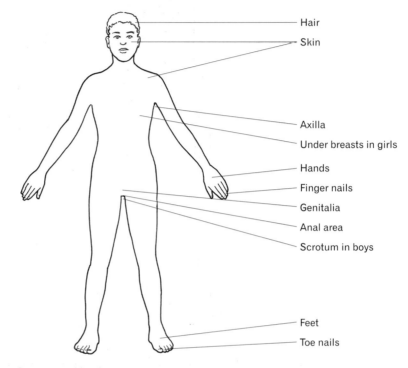

— Hair
— Skin
— Axilla
— Under breasts in girls
— Hands
— Finger nails
— Genitalia
— Anal area
— Scrotum in boys
— Feet
— Toe nails

Areas for personal hygiene

Social relationships

Adolescents may experience some difficulty in relating to other people, such as parents, teachers or anyone else in authority. Others may find it hard to maintain communication with peers and feel like an outsider. Some adolescents may show signs of:

- *anti-social behaviour* – the adolescent shows signs of disobedience and aggression. In most cases, this may be a step towards achieving independence, and may be a temporary phase. In some cases, if this behaviour persists, it may just be the sign of a more complicated problem. Additional support from the GP or a counsellor may be necessary
- *isolation* – the adolescent may isolate themselves or be isolated by their peers. This is very painful for the adolescent who may change the way she looks, her clothes or her lifestyle in order to fit back in with her peers.

Emotional support

Providing support with regard to relationships is an important part of caring for adolescents. It includes the following aspects.

Information about sexual relationships

Adolescents feel self-conscious discussing sexual relationships in the presence of adults, such as their parents. However, they often have no difficulty in discussing sexual conquests with their peers. It is important that they receive information and advice with regard to:

- *sexual relationships* – adolescents who are sexually active may develop a **sexually-transmitted disease (STD)**, an infection such as gonorrhoea passed on through unprotected intercourse with an infected partner (see page 124). The importance of contraception needs to be explained, with its benefits – protection from disease and unwanted pregnancy (see *Teenage pregnancy*, page 124)

- *masturbation* – in adolescence, boys and girls become aware of the sexual aspects of their body. The exploration of their sexual awareness may be through masturbation – creating sexual arousal, and sometimes orgasm, by caressing one's own genital areas. For most children, masturbation starts well before puberty, as many young children find pleasure in handling their genitals. They should not be told off as this promotes guilt. Children and adolescents should be encouraged to have a positive view of their bodies.

Boundaries and adult support

As part of their growing independence, adolescents still need boundaries for acceptable behaviour as testing these is part of the process of growing up. The adolescent without these can feel insecure as they have no solid guideline against which to exercise their independence. For example, most adolescents may argue about the time they have to be home after an evening out. If this restraint was absent, there would be no growing sense of independence. In adulthood, these boundaries are often viewed in a positive light, whereas during adolescence they are a cause for friction. Discussing what is sensible, and not being swayed by what others are allowed to do, is a way of meeting the needs of both adults and adolescents.

Boundaries of adult support are necessary requirements for the health and safety of the adolescent, who can be vulnerable and need protection.

Affection and strong relationships

Although adolescents can be difficult and moody, they still need to be loved and to feel secure in their rapidly changing world. They still respond to routines because this is important for their growing independence. The emphasis is on their outward appearance, behaviour and fitting in with peers so adults are expected to accept this preoccupation. Parents find this difficult – their loving cuddly son or daughter suddenly does not want to be kissed goodbye in front of school friends.

Being available to discuss and respond to issues is part of giving affection and supporting the adolescent through one of the most difficult periods of their lives.

LIFE EVENTS

On the whole, adolescents cope well with predicted changes. They see these as part of their progression to adulthood and to independence. Unpredictable events, such as the death of a parent or a divorce, are obviously much harder to cope with. This is due to the many physical changes that teenagers are experiencing and the effect this may have on their sense of security. Any additional negative experiences can be particularly difficult to manage.

Table 8.2 gives examples of predictable and unpredictable events which may affect adolescents.

Predictable events	Unpredictable events
Going to secondary school	Premature disability/disease
Friendships and being part of a peer group	Breakdown in relationships
Career aspirations and progression	Drug misuse
Being part of a family group	Pregnancy
	Death or divorce in the family

Table 8.2 Predictable and unpredictable events in adolescence

SPECIAL AND ADDITIONAL NEEDS

Special needs which may arise during adolescence may be a result of:

- eating disorders
- drug misuse
- sexually-transmitted disease
- teenage pregnancy
- smoking and alcohol.

Eating disorders

An eating disorder is a serious disruption of a person's eating habits, which affects their health and well-being. The two most common eating disorders are:

- *anorexia nervosa* – occurs when a person either refuses to eat or, if she does eat, she will then make herself sick in order to remove the food, or take large doses of laxatives
- *bulimia nervosa* – involves eating vast quantities of food (bingeing) and then vomiting the food in the secrecy of the toilet.

These conditions are motivated by a false view of being overweight or by a fear of becoming overweight, and the need to lose weight. They commonly affect adolescent girls, but boys are also affected.

The girl (or boy), who becomes obsessive about food, views her body with disgust. She discovers very quickly how to hide her disorder. She may make a great show of eating but either finds an excuse to throw it away, or goes straight to the toilet to induce vomiting. She will weigh herself several times a day and will get distressed if she puts on weight. These eating disorders may even cause the person to starve herself to death. She needs medical supervision and treatment. In severe cases this may involve hospitalisation. It is an extremely distressing time for her family who may use all manner of strategies to help her to eat. The girl herself has to make a conscious decision to put on weight. Unless she does, no treatment will be successful.

Drug misuse

Drug misuse is the term used to describe taking illegal drugs, such as heroin, marijuana, cocaine, amphetamines, diethylamide (LSD) and Ecstasy in different forms. It also includes solvent abuse, which involves young people inhaling fumes from solvents such as glues and aerosols, and the misuse of legally prescribed drugs.

There are a number of reasons why young people experiment with drugs, such as:

- peer pressure
- curiosity
- to relieve stress and anxiety
- availability
- having no regard or concern for their safety.

Whatever the reason, drug misuse has a damaging effect on the body. Medical treatment is available through the National Health Service and is a priority concern for the Government and for local authorities.

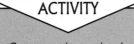

ACTIVITY

The Government has produced a document called **Tackling Drugs Together – To Build a Better Britain** (1998). Borrow a copy from the library and discuss the main issues involved.

Sexually-transmitted diseases

These are diseases such as genital herpes, non-specific urethritis, syphilis and HIV (Human Immunodeficiency Virus – AIDS). Such diseases are passed on through unprotected sex. (There are also other ways in which HIV is contracted, such as through the use of dirty or shared needles and syringes, through infected blood transfusions, and via the placenta from the mother to the unborn foetus).

Sex education is essential for adolescents. Clear explanation of the dangers of unprotected sex and other information and advice should always be available. GP surgeries, libraries, schools and all public service areas should have some information with regard to contraception.

Should sexually transmitted diseases be contracted, they are treated in genito-urinary clinics where advice and treatment is free and confidential.

Teenage pregnancy

Teenage pregnancy strictly speaking refers to a pregnancy in any girl in her teenage years; in practice it is used to describe a pregnancy in a girl who is still a minor, i.e. under 16 and of statutory school age.

A girl under 16 who is pregnant will face the choice either to have an abortion or to give birth to the baby, and then, whether the baby can be adopted or kept by the girl. Whatever choice is made, a great deal of support is needed.

If the girl decides to keep the baby, support can be given by:

- helping the girl to develop practical baby-care skills
- providing day care so that the young mother can return to school to continue her education
- providing home tutoring until she can return to school
- providing medical support through the GP, midwife and health visitor.

Smoking and alcohol

Smoking

Smoking amongst young people, especially girls, is on the increase. It is known to have damaging effects on the body, such as causing lung and heart disease. It should be recognised that smoking is an addiction to nicotine and that giving up smoking can be very difficult.

KEY POINT

Adolescents under the age of 16 are not allowed to buy cigarettes, but this does not seem to deter them.

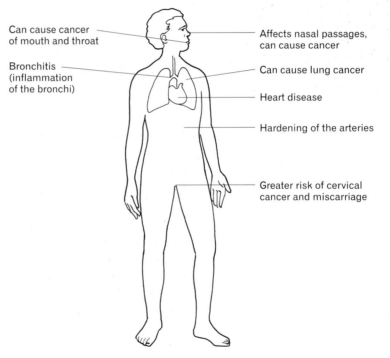

Can cause cancer of mouth and throat

Bronchitis (inflammation of the bronchi)

Affects nasal passages, can cause cancer

Can cause lung cancer

Heart disease

Hardening of the arteries

Greater risk of cervical cancer and miscarriage

Physical effects of smoking on the body

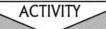
ACTIVITY

Visit your local library, health centre and chemist and collect any information that is available about smoking and alcohol. Look in particular for information that is aimed at teenagers.

Alcohol

Alcohol is the result of the fermentation process of yeasts on fruits and cereals. It can be drunk as beer and wine. Spirits, such as gin, vodka and whisky, are produced through distilling alcohol. Alcohol can have serious effects on the body, particularly if consumed in excess.

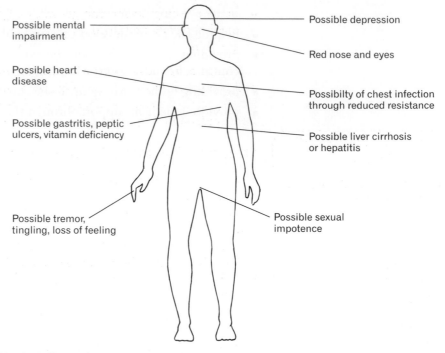

Physical effects of alcohol on the body

Health education has an important role to play in offering free information and advice to young people on the adverse effects of smoking and alcohol.

SOURCES OF SUPPORT

Support is available through family and friends, as well as through the school, the local education authority, the Youth Service and voluntary groups.

Rights and responsibilities

The Children Act 1989 supports the rights of children and young people. Adolescents also have some rights and responsibilities laid down in law. These include the following:

- at 10 a child has reached the age of criminal responsibility
- at 12 a child can purchase a pet
- at 14 a child can go unaccompanied to see a film which is classified PG (Parental Guidance)
- at 16 a young person can buy cigarettes, marry with their parents' consent, give consent for medical treatment
- at 17 a young person can live away from home without their parents' consent, learn to drive

- at 18 a young person can get married without parent's consent, can buy alcohol legally and drink in public houses, can vote in local and national elections.

Adolescence is a time of growing and changing, which can lead to difficulties and problems. However, there is much that the adolescent and the parents can do to help make the changes as smooth as possible. Good communication, understanding, sympathy, and tolerance are needed on both sides.

Organisations which offer support in adolescence

Action on Smoking and Health (ASH), 109 Gloucester Place, London W1H 4EJ

Alcohol Concern, Waterbridge House, 32–36 Loman Street, London SE1 0EE

British Heart Foundation, 14 Fitzhardinge Street, London W1H 4DH

Childline, Freepost 1111, London N1 0BR

Children's Society, Edward Rudolf House, Margery Street, London WC1X 0JL

Health Education Authority, Hamilton House, Mabeldon Place, London WC1H 9TX

Release (Drugs and Legal Helpline), 169 Commercial Street, London E1 6BW

Shaftesbury Society, Shaftesbury House, 2a Amity Grove, London SW20 0LH

Shelter, 88 Old Street, London EC1V 9HU

Youth Clubs UK, 11 St Bride Street, London EC4A 4AS

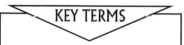

KEY TERMS

You need to know the meaning of the following words and phrases. Go back through the chapter to make sure that you understand them.

adolescence
drug misuse
eating disorder
primary sexual characteristics
puberty
secondary sexual characteristics
sexually-transmitted disease

Caring for adults

PREVIEW

Adulthood is the longest period of the lifespan. It covers a range of changes over approximately 47 years. This chapter will enable you to develop your understanding of:

- Growth and development
- Basic needs
- Care issues
- Life events
- Special and additional needs
- Sources of support.

Adulthood is officially recognised as beginning at the age of 18 years when the young person becomes eligible to vote, and extends to 65 years of age and beyond. For convenience, and for the purposes of this book, adulthood ends with retirement at 65 years of age, and old age begins (covered in Chapter 10). However, it should be remembered that there is no sudden transition at 65 – it is a gradual process. Most people are still active members of society at 65 and continue to be so for many years, although the process of ageing is increasing its pace and many will find themselves in need of care later.

A number of aspects characterise adulthood, as the individual moves from the relative dependence of their early years to a place of responsibility and independence. Being an adult should enable a person to take control of their lives by making their own decisions and choices.

GROWTH AND DEVELOPMENT

Adulthood involves many transitions. There are three distinct age phases as summarised in Table 9.1.

Phase	Examples of characteristics
Young adulthood 18–40 years (approx.)	• Usually in good physical health • Working towards employment, making career choices • Forming relationships with view to long-term partnership or marriage • Parenting – setting up family life, i.e. having children
Mid-adulthood 40–65 years (approx.)	• Usually a time of re-evaluation of their lives • Some decline in sensory abilities, co-ordination and reaction time • Varying degrees of physical health • Some adults peak in their careers during this time • Women in particular begin to experience hormonal changes, i.e. the menopause
Late adulthood 65+ years (see Chapter 10)	• A time of adjustment – retirement from employment • Effects of ageing are present in the physical, intellectual, social and emotional aspects of growth • Relationship changes, i.e. within family, children are now adults

Table 9.1 Phases of adulthood and their characteristics

> ## KEY POINT
>
> The main features of physical development in adulthood include the following.
>
> • Maximum height is attained and strength peaks at about the age of 30.
>
> • Sexual potency reaches its peak in late adolescence for men, and in the mid-twenties for women.
>
> • Many women normally cease menstruation at sometime between 40 and 50 years of age.

Physical development

During adulthood, people reach the peak of their development and physical performance. Skeletal growth ends in early adulthood and physiologically body mechanisms are working efficiently. From the age of 30, ageing begins and can affect some of these physiological processes which begin to slow down. There is an increase of adipose or fatty tissue on different parts of the body and some people begin to put on weight which they find difficult to lose.

There is a clear stage of development for women from approximately their late thirties extending into their mid-fifties because they are approaching the **menopause**, which means the end to their reproductive function. During the menopause, the ovaries reduce the production of the hormone oestrogen and menstruation becomes irregular and eventually ceases. Some women can suffer side effects such as headaches, tension, mood swings, hot flushes and osteoporosis (see the diagram on page 136).

Intellectual and cognitive development

Intellectual and cognitive abilities develop throughout the lifespan, although in some cases memory is affected as brain cells die. There are a number of issues which present themselves with regard to the adult's intellectual and cognitive development. These are as follows.

Adult thought and cognitive skills

Adults in middle age can and do continue to learn new skills. This learning should be supported with much encouragement, as one of the blocks to their

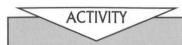

ACTIVITY

Visit the local library and make a list of all the courses which are available to adult students. If you are attending college, make enquiries about which courses are available for mature students.

learning may be a lack of confidence. Positive encouragement and reminding the adult that they have valuable life experience is essential. These experiences should enhance the adult's reasoning and problem-solving skills.

Educational opportunities

Lifelong learning is a process whereby a person's educational needs can be met in the adult years. Many colleges, schools and adult education centres offer courses to appeal to mature students. Some courses offer formal qualifications leading to a degree, while others offer the opportunity to learn a foreign language, gain computer skills or study a variety of other subjects and learn new skills.

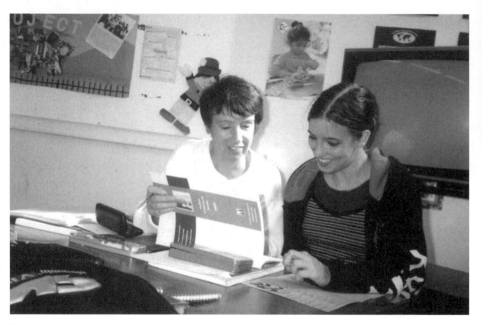

Now I have time to study: many adults gain in confidence and fulfil long-held ambitions through lifelong learning

Using television and video as a means of gaining information can stimulate the learning process leading to further reading and research. However, television may have the reverse effect. Some adults may be content to sit in front of the television for long periods and block out their surroundings.

Career, work and age

Progressing into middle age, adults may be moving to the peak of a career chosen in early adulthood, earning more money, building an affluent lifestyle and rising to a management position in their place of work. On the other hand, some adults may have faced a pattern of redundancy and unemployment. For some this may be a launch pad for a positive change in career direction.

The result of work is the financial reward and income which enables the individual to choose the lifestyle they wish to follow. Adults without employment do not have these choices. They may often have difficulty in maintaining a minimum basic lifestyle. They are denied the opportunities which are available to them in the world of work such as developing new skills and reinforcing existing ones.

Emotional and personality development

There are different times in adulthood in which identity, love and work are features. This may involve learning from others such as the family, peers and colleagues. Young adults may observe and watch how individuals contribute to a variety of situations, such as the management of people at work, relationships with colleagues, friendships, partnerships, hobbies, sport and leisure, finance, employment possibilities and career aspirations. Through observation, a young adult may test the outside world to 'see what works for them'.

In the analysis of development by Erikson (1968), he reveals the different psychological and social stages and transitions of the adult life between 20 and 65 years of age. In the eight-stage progression shown in the table on page 68, there are two stages which apply to adults. They are:

- *Stage 6 (18–30s): Intimacy versus isolation* The character of the adult has been formed, but the person's identity may be developed further by sharing a relationship with another person. Building a strong relationship with another will involve identifying strengths and weaknesses and working together. In the event of not building a relationship and commitment to another, the person may become isolated and feel left out. This may lead to the person becoming self-absorbed in their own activities and interests.

- *Stage 7 (20s–60s): **Generativity** versus **stagnation*** Approaching middle age leads either to generativity or stagnation.
  - Generativity means that the adult is concerned for others and life beyond the immediate family. They may be involved with community and voluntary work, trying to make the world a better place to live in.
  - Stagnation means that the adult becomes increasingly concerned with themselves and their lifestyle. They are constantly pre-occupied with their personal needs and can become fixed in their views and attitudes.

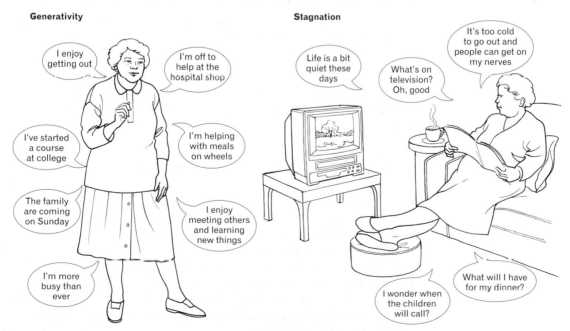

Generativity and stagnation

It is important to recognise that adults face a number of changing circumstances and may balance a number of social roles in daily living, for example, wife, mother, nurse, aunt, daughter or husband, teacher, uncle, father, brother.

CASE STUDY

James

James is 24 years old. He has been travelling around the world but has now returned to live in London. He has started work as a clerical officer for a local council. He lives in a bed sitter and finds it difficult to make friends. His parents have retired to Devon, and he visits them once a month. His old university acquaintances have made new friends and some are in steady relationships.

1 Can you identify James in Erikson's stage of intimacy versus isolation (page 131)?

2 How would you support James?

3 What advice would you give him?

Social development and building relationships

Social development in adults has an important role. It involves building and maintaining relationships and coping with changes in family life which include:

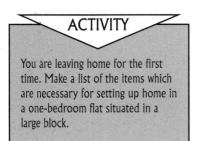

ACTIVITY

You are leaving home for the first time. Make a list of the items which are necessary for setting up home in a one-bedroom flat situated in a large block.

- *leaving home* – after the search for an identity which takes place during adolescence, the majority of young adults find themselves concerned with getting their lives in order so that they gain financial and emotional independence. Many will either have left home or will be thinking about it. Leaving home is quite a traumatic experience, as it is the first step into an adult life. However, this may be counter-balanced by the excitement of building a new life

- *making a new home* – the young adult will either try to make a replica of his family home or break free entirely and create something very different. Either way, most adults will feel homesick at times, mainly through feelings of insecurity and the fear of change. In time, if they do not give in to these fears, young adults will learn to come to terms with their changed situation. They will accept their new accommodation as 'home' and be glad to be there

- *parental attitudes* – the reaction of parents to the growing independence of their adult children may affect the situation. Most parents who genuinely want their child to gain independence will offer support and help where necessary, and will not try to prevent their son or daughter from leaving home. In fact, if parents can see this period as an opportunity to spend more time with each other rather than as the loss of their child, they will have a far healthier attitude to what is, after all, a natural progression from adolescence to adulthood

● *forming relationships* – by the time they are in their twenties, many people are in the process of forming a steady relationship, whether heterosexual or homosexual. In a sexual relationship, the couple have the option of living together or separately, getting engaged or getting married. Some adults choose to be single while others remain single because they have not formed a permanent relationship. Networking in friendships is a strategy used by some adults who wish to maintain contact with a number of old friends and to set up social occasions when they can meet regularly.

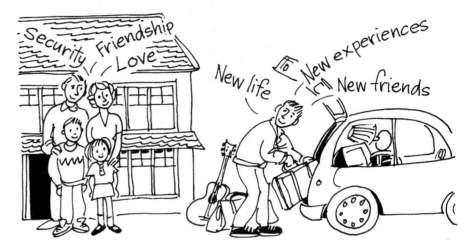

Moving towards independence

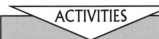
BASIC NEEDS

The basic needs which affect adulthood reflect the ways in which the adult life changes and develops.

Emotional needs

Adults have emotional needs, which may involve selecting and learning to live with a partner, sexual relationships, starting a family and rearing children.

Learning to live with a partner

Partnerships may be permanent or short-term. Having met a partner, the relationship-building process begins. Will they be compatible and be able to accommodate each other's personality traits? Will they be able to settle into a life together? – early adulthood may be viewed by some as a period of freedom, i.e. living life to the full before settling down, while others may have already established a relationship, set up home and are rearing children.

Maintaining a strong and positive relationship with a partner is, in most cases, successful, but in some cases the relationship can break down. There are a number of reasons why relationships break down, including incompatibility, involvement with others outside the partnership and domestic violence.

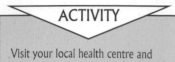

ACTIVITY

Visit your local health centre and find out about the different methods of contraception available.

Sexual relationships

Every adult has sexual needs and a sexual identity. Sexual relationships are an important part of life. Sexual intercourse can be mutually enjoyable for a consenting couple. It can enhance and support a loving and secure partnership. Most adults have attitudes and views about a sexual relationship which should always be respected even when they are different to those of others.

However, when a couple have differing attitudes about sex, this may lead to difficulties. Films and television heighten people's expectations, but the reality of a couple's life can be completely different. When difficulties arise, the couple should be encouraged to discuss them with each other and wherever possible to look for a solution to the problem.

In some cases, one adult may have decided to have a sexual relationship with a person outside the partnership. This is often a very difficult issue for the other partner to cope with. Sometimes it can lead to breakdown in relationships.

Consenting adults should always ensure that they use effective contraception and use condoms to ensure safe sex.

Not all consenting sexual relationships are heterosexual. Remember that homosexual relationships are equally satisfying and secure. The rights, views and beliefs of people in homosexual relationships should be respected.

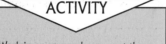

ACTIVITY

Work in groups and carry out the following tasks.

a) Make a list of the different aspects of care, which support physical, emotional, intellectual, cultural and social development, that parents use in caring for their children at 3 years, 10 years and 16 years of age.

b) Review the list and compare the methods used for the different age groups.

c) Prioritise the list of methods, giving reasons.

Starting a family and rearing children

Making a decision to have a baby together is viewed by some couples as the first step to a more permanent relationship. The baby is regarded as the way in which the relationship can be developed and strengthened.

Bringing up young children, caring and supporting them as they grow and develop through the different stages of life can be demanding. Growing children need time, energy and attention.

Many couples may work together to meet their children's different needs, while others may leave the responsibility to just one parent. This can often lead to friction, as the parent taking most of the responsibility can feel resentful. Lone or single parents usually take sole and full responsibility for the rearing of their children without the support of a partner.

The role of the adult changes as their children become teenagers. It becomes the task of assisting their teenage children to develop into responsible and happy adults. This may require setting boundaries for growing teenagers, which are necessary for them to cope with any difficulties that they may be experiencing.

Supporting and encouraging teenagers towards adulthood is not a easy task. Many parents need support from others during this time, either in a voluntary, informal capacity, such as through family and friends, or through a professional counselling agency, such as Relate.

Maintaining a home and establishing a standard of living

Most adults will set up a home of their own and maintain it, providing a safe, secure, positive and healthy environment. This is an important factor in achieving their adult independence.

- *Establishing and maintaining an economic standard of living* involves adopting strategies to support the present lifestyle and, wherever possible, saving for the future. The scope of such actions will be dependent on income.

- *The type of home and the standard of living* may be determined by the salary of the adults living there. This will differ in most cases. In some, it will be affected by social class and status in society, with professional and upper-class adults owning bigger houses and cars. People who are working class, unskilled workers, the jobless or unemployed and those receiving benefit will often struggle to survive in smaller accommodation.

Career and employment needs

Making career and employment choices may be based on learning and education experiences. By their late twenties, men and women may be married (or have made a decision to stay single), living in a relationship with another person, divorced or separated or may be concentrating on developing a career, setting up a lifestyle and building up their home life. People at this age are usually active, energetic and ambitious.

As adults get older, career and employment needs and preferences may change. This may be related to a reduction in work opportunities due to budget cuts, for health reasons, or a wish for a change of lifestyle.

CASE STUDY

Jeremy and Margaret

Jeremy and Margaret are in their thirties. They are very successful in their jobs – Jeremy is a stockbroker and Margaret is a marketing executive. They do not have children. One day they realise that middle age is 'just around the corner'. They are beginning to feel that life is passing them by as Jeremy has been recently passed over for promotion by a younger man.

1 Do you think that they are over-reacting with regard to their age?

2 Look at a selection of recruitment pages in newspapers. What ages are mentioned?

Social, leisure and recreation needs

Most adults enjoy meeting and socialising with others in a number of ways, such as meeting in the pub, going to church or joining a group to pursue special interests. Some adults are interested in community life and become actively involved with assisting others, for example, by joining the local council, supporting charities or self-help groups. Other adults enjoy different forms of recreation, such as holidays, going to the gym, swimming, walking, music or taking an interest in the environment.

Social, leisure and recreation needs are often based on the amount of choice which is available. In some cases these activities are highly dependent on income, with the poorer, low-income families being limited in their choices.

Physical and psychological changes of middle age

Physical and psychological needs may occur as a result of ageing. Adults need to accept that the ageing process is occurring, that it is inevitable and that it will not go away. Some people suffer from a mid-life crisis when they are confronted by the fact that they are growing old and try to avoid the implications.

Women begin experience the symptoms of the menopause as they grow older. Some men and women suffer early symptoms of ageing such as hair loss or baldness, grey hair, failing eyesight, as well as various aches and pains.

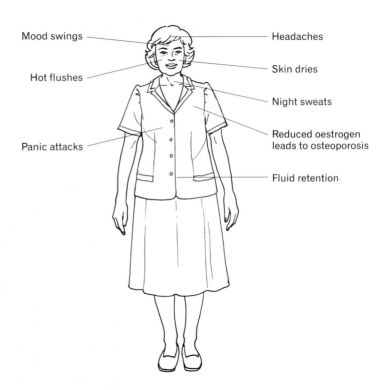

Mood swings

Hot flushes

Panic attacks

Headaches

Skin dries

Night sweats

Reduced oestrogen leads to osteoporosis

Fluid retention

The signs and symptoms of the menopause

It should be a time when adults begin to enjoy life in a new way. On the other hand, people can become dissatisfied and unhappy with how they have spent their lives. To cope with any destructive feelings which may result, the adults concerned need to be able to accept themselves for who they are. They should be encouraged to look at what they have achieved in their lives and to learn to be reasonably satisfied rather than worrying about what they have not done.

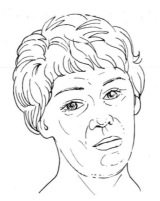 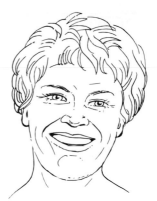

What have I achieved?
Nothing much. The children left home because
they could not stand it any longer.
What is left for me now? I feel so inadequate
and helpless.

I have achieved something… I have a loving
family. I have the opportunity to seek fresh
direction. I have started a college course
and made new friends.

Views of personal achievements

Caring for older parents

Later adulthood brings with it a role reversal. As their children are becoming independent, some older adults find themselves providing care for their older parents. Giving the necessary support and care, in whatever way possible, becomes a priority.

Trying to balance this issue within the context of middle age can be difficult. Adults have their own needs and demands which they often have to balance with the needs of their parents. In some cases, older people find it difficult to 'let go' of their adult children and become too demanding.

These are issues which families have to work through together. Contact with services involved with older people may provide a valuable means of support to both adults and their parents.

Health needs

Between the ages of 45 and 60, the previously healthy adult may begin to suffer from ill health. At this stage of adulthood, the death rate starts to increase, largely due to cancer, heart disease and strokes, as well as respiratory and circulatory disorders. Health education campaigns can play an important part by encouraging healthy diets and regular exercise. The likelihood of developing illnesses can be reduced by eating a healthy diet and by taking regular exercise. If these lifestyle changes take place during middle age, they will help to prevent existing medical conditions from getting any worse.

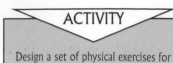

ACTIVITY

Design a set of physical exercises for a group of 50-year-old men and women. What exercises would you recommend?

Physical exercise may have many benefits. It is possible to select a range of exercises to meet the individual needs of each person. Exercising should always reflect a person's physical level of attainment and their lifestyle. Adults should be encouraged to have a medical check up with their GP before embarking on an exercise programme.

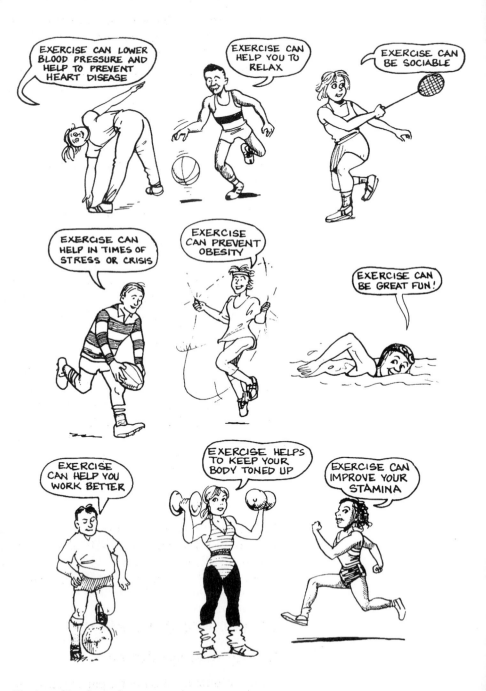

The benefits of exercise

CARE ISSUES

Carers and care workers become involved in supporting adults when a special need arises. This is usually at times of ill health, accident, redundancy, domestic violence and problems with relationships.

Social relationships

Issues which relate to social relationships may involve the following.

Supporting adults who want to start a family

Carers can help by offering information which will include advice with regard to a healthy diet, vitamins or reducing the intake of alcohol. These are factors which may increase the likelihood of conception. Encouraging the couple to visit their GP, stopping the use of contraception and monitoring the woman's ovulation dates for her most fertile time for conception would be useful strategies.

Supporting parents and families

Some young parents find child-rearing stressful. Carers can be supportive by being available to listen, offering advice and child-care, and looking after the children to give the parents a break.

Parenting teenagers may be difficult and there may be times when parents feel that they are not coping. Carers can have an important role by being available to listen and by giving reassurance at a trying time.

During middle age, adults may have teenage children to care for and they often have the additional responsibility of their own ageing parents. Carers can support the family by exploring ways in which the older parent can be given additional support and care.

Employment advice

Some adults may have needs with regard to employment. The carer has a role in supporting adults with employment needs. When a person has become unemployed, or has been made redundant, then support is necessary. Giving advice, information about job clubs, benefits and the writing of job applications are important aspects of giving additional support and care. Carers should be available to talk about possible career aspirations and to encourage the adult to visit the local adult education centres to check what courses are on offer.

Financial support

Working with families who are experiencing financial problems needs a sensitive and caring approach. Carers should listen to difficulties and, wherever possible, arrange for specialist counselling which is available through the local Citizen's Advice Bureau.

EMOTIONAL SUPPORT

Empty nest syndrome

Many middle-aged parents, particularly mothers, feel that they have lost a parental role and can feel useless when a child leaves home. This is due to the fact that they have not considered themselves in any other role. This is called empty nest syndrome! Carers can have a supportive role in ensuring that such a parent is directed to information and advice with regard to opportunities for community involvement, possible courses and new hobbies.

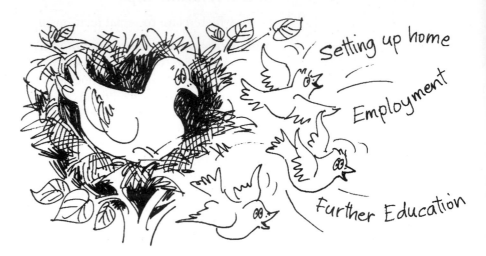

Empty nest syndrome

Adults with psychological needs

Middle age is the time of life when men and women often wonder what they have achieved in life. These thoughts may lead to feelings of guilt and depression. This can be referred to as the 'mid-life crisis', a term which reflects the depth of feeling about middle age.

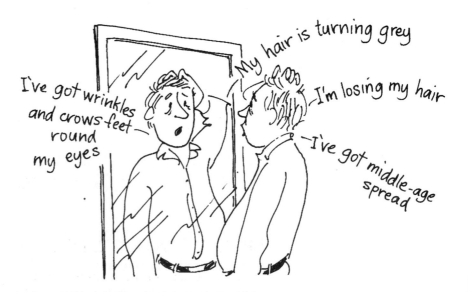

Help! I'm middle-aged

ACTIVITY

In groups, discuss and decide the strategies of care which would be necessary in the following cases.

a) Michael is 24 years old. He lives in a bedsit in a town centre. He works in a bookshop and recently, during a skiing holiday, he fell and broke his ankle. His parents live in Africa, so they are not able to care for him. He has friends who live nearby and they have offered to do some shopping.

b) Harry and Mavis are in their early sixties. They live in a large detached house in the country. They have three dogs and two cats. Harry suffers from dementia and often forgets what he is doing and wanders off. Mavis has coped with the situation but recently she has also begun to feel unwell, complaining of chest pains and tiredness. They have no children and rely on neighbours for help with the pets, i.e. walking the dogs.

c) Josh and Salma Patel have three children, aged 2, 4 and 6. Recently they have been told that their oldest child Abdul has leukaemia. They are devastated and feel helpless. They have a large extended family. Josh has three brothers and his parents are still alive but live in Pakistan. Salma's mother lives nearby with her brother and his family.

One response to the mid-life crisis is to try to recapture lost youth, rather than accepting and enjoying the middle years. Adults may feel certain regrets: perhaps they were not as successful at work as they had hoped, or possibly they may feel bored with their personal relationships and long to recapture some romance and excitement.

Some adults may embark on new relationships. This may result in the breakdown of existing long-term partnerships. These relationships may be with much younger people, in an attempt to make the person feel younger.

Whatever the psychological condition, carers can offer support and listen to the needs of the adult. Where there is an underlying psychiatric disorder, specialist help may be necessary.

Women at this age need support and encouragement to extend their horizons and to use this period of their lives as an opportunity to develop new interests, such as adult education classes, a new career, new hobbies and leisure pursuits.

Assistance with long-term or short-term ill health

As adulthood progresses, the possibility of ill health increases. There are many practical ways in which carers and care workers can support adults. The measure of support will depend on the severity of the disease, disorder or disability. For example, if the adult has had a stroke and is paralysed, the different strategies of care such as helping with toileting, feeding and maintaining their general health and well-being will be paramount.

In addition to giving practical support, carers and care workers can arrange links with self-help groups such as Mencap, Backup and Relate which provide information and advice.

LIFE EVENTS

Examples of predictable and unpredictable events that may occur during adulthood are given in Table 9.2.

Predictable events	Unpredictable events
Completion of education	Ill health
Employment	Disability
Setting up a home	Bereavement
Steady relationship	Unemployment/redundancy
Starting a family	Homelessness
	Divorce
	Poverty

Table 9.2 Examples of predictable and unpredictable events in adulthood

SPECIAL AND ADDITIONAL NEEDS

There are times during adulthood when adults will have a special or additional need which requires consistent care and support.

Divorce and separation

The break-up of a relationship is a very painful experience especially when there are children involved. It may be a short-term break-up such as a separation, or it may become permanant.

Divorce is legal and permanent separation. In some cases, a divorce can become a battleground for financial reasons and for the custody of children. Divorce is a time of anxiety and distress for all concerned. It is second only to bereavement on the stress scale. In some people it may cause psychological and physical ill health. Conciliation services provide support which enable the couple to try to settle their differences. Their aim is to help the couple to part as amicably as possible.

Infertility

Infertility is the inability of a woman to conceive or of a man to induce conception. It is a distressing experience for both partners. Possible causes of infertility include:

- inactive sperm in the semen
- the pituitary gland producing too much prolactin which leads to impotence in the male and infertility in the woman
- the man failing to have an erection
- fallopian tubes being blocked
- ovaries not producing eggs
- mucus lining in the vagina becoming thick and so sperm cannot enter.

A couple often expect to conceive a baby as soon as they make the decision to start a family. They feel disappointed and frustrated when conception fails to happen. They may need specialised counselling. Discussing their infertility with a GP or a gynaecologist will give them the opportunity to find out the cause of their inability to conceive. In some cases medical treatment may be necessary, such as unblocking the fallopian tubes or treating any pelvic infection.

Domestic violence

Domestic violence is abuse which occurs within a partnership or family. It involves power and control by one person within the relationship. One partner uses physical, emotional, economic, sexual or psychological means to exercise control over the other.

Domestic violence is a criminal offence and may take place in *any* relationship regardless of race, class, culture or religion. In the majority of cases, the violence is carried out by a man against a woman. The woman may be physically injured but will feel that, in some ways, she has been responsible for the violent outburst. She may try to cover up for her partner. Where domestic violence is suspected, it should be reported to the police. The woman will need specialist support from agencies such as Women's Aid.

Domestic violence against men can also occur, as women have been known to be violent and threatening to their partners. However, this is not as prevalent as violence towards women.

ACTIVITY

In groups, find out which agencies are available to offer support to patients with cancer and to their families. What sort of support do they offer?

Disease, disability and death

Life-threatening disease

Life-threatening disease can take many forms, of which cancer is the most common. For an adult to discover that they have a form of malignant cancer, i.e. cancer which spreads to other parts of the body, can be very frightening and distressing to both the person concerned, their family and friends

Medical treatment should be discussed with the adult affected and their family. Any distressing symptoms should be identified and nursing and caring strategies set up. For example the side effects of chemotherapy can include vomiting, loss of appetite, diarrhoea, loss of hair and vulnerability to infection. Supporting care for a frail person may involve providing small but nutritious meals as well as assisting with hygiene and toileting routines.

In such cases there are support groups and agencies such as Backup which offer assistance to patients and their families. The groups usually consist of those who have been through similar experiences. This type of support can be a valuable means of helping the individual to come to terms with disease.

During their lifespan, adults may be parents of children with life-threatening disease and illness. Support offered to such parents is discussed in Chapter 7, page 107–8, 109.

Accidents which cause long-term disability

When accidents occur, they can be distressing to any adult. When the long-term effects of the accident bring permanent disability, such as paralysis of a limb, the impact can be even more devastating. It may lead to changes in lifestyle. For example the adult may not be able to work, causing a sharp reduction in income.

Accidents can occur in a number of contexts, such as a serious car accident, an accident in the home or an injury whilst at work.

Death and bereavement

In some cases, illness and disease, accidents and injury can lead to death. During adulthood, people may experience the death of a baby, child, partner, mother, father, close relative or friend. There are different ways of supporting the bereaved person to cope with the event. This is discussed in Chapter 10 (page 164).

Redundancy

Redundancy (the loss of paid employment), for whatever reason, may be a difficult and painful experience for any adult. The methods used to issue the redundancy can be distressing, leaving the person concerned feeling depressed and rejected.

By law, employers are required to issue a notice of redundancy and discuss the terms of any redundancy payment with the employee. This does not diminish the negative feelings which the adult may have, such as:

- anger and anxiety due to loss of income
- a sense of rejection and concerns about future employment
- a sense of helplessness, especially if they have a home and a family to care for.

Those who face redundancy need to be supported and helped to overcome the sense of rejection. Redundancy should be recognised as a loss and that there is a grieving process involved, which may take some time to overcome. Allowing the adult to talk through their frustrations will help them to face the future and to see the options available to them. They may use the experience to return to study, to change their career or to develop new skills.

CASE STUDY

Patrick

Patrick has worked in care management for 25 years. He works in a rest home, for 30 older clients, which is situated in a coastal town. One day, the home owner tells Patrick that the business has been sold and that the new owners are extending the premises to cater for 75 older clients. Patrick is excited at the prospect. He meets the new owners and feels optimistic about the future. When the extensions are finished, however, the new owners tell Patrick that they feel he lacks sufficient experience to manage the home and they issue him with a redundancy notice.

1　How would you react if you were Patrick?

2　Discuss the actions of the home owners.

3　How would you support Patrick and what advice would you give him?

4　Are there any support agencies that Patrick can be referred to?

SOURCES OF SUPPORT

There are many organisations available to support adults with a variety of needs. Social support may come through friends and family. Medical and professional support is available through various career and employment agencies and through the National Health Service.

Organisations available to support adults

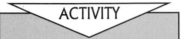

ACTIVITY

There are a number of organisations which exist to support adults. Review this list and add some organisations which you have researched. Find out what sort of support each organisation gives, and to whom.

Backup, 3 Bath Place, Rivington Street, London EC2A 3JR

Equal Opportunities Commission, Overseas House, Quay Street, Manchester M33 3HN

Gingerbread, 16 Clerkenwell Court, London EC1R OAA

Health Education Authority, Hamilton House, Mabledon Place, London WC1H 9TX

Low Pay Unit, 9 Berkeley Street, London W1H 8BY

Mencap, 123 Golden Lane, London EC1Y 0RT

National Association of Citizens Advice Bureaux, Myddleton House, 115–123 Pentonville Road, London N1 0LZ

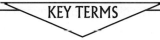

KEY TERMS

You need to know the meaning of the following words and phrases. Go back through the chapter to make sure that you understand them.

adulthood
divorce
domestic violence
generativity
infertility
lifelong learning
menopause
stagnation

National Council for Voluntary Organisations, Regent's Wharf, 8 All Saints Street, London N1 9RL

Parentline UK, Endway House, The Endway, Hadleigh, Essex SS7 2AN

Relate, Herbert Gray College, Little Church Street, Rugby, Warwickshire CV21 3AP

Samaritans, 10 The Grove, Slough SL1 1QP

Women's Health, 52 Featherstone Street, London EC1Y 8RT

Women's Aid Federation, PO Box 391, Bristol BS99 7WS

Caring for older people

PREVIEW

The care of older people covers a range of needs which may develop during an individual's growth and development through the lifespan. Most of the needs of this age relate to the ageing process. This chapter will enable you to develop your understanding of:

- Growth and development
- Basic needs
- Care issues
- Life events
- Special and additional needs
- Sources of support.

The process of ageing is very gradual and in fact begins at birth. During a life time the individual will grow and develop in many ways, including physical, intellectual, cognitive, emotional, social and cultural. All these have been mentioned in previous chapters. The 'elderly' stage is the final part of the lifespan. Although this stage is identified with retirement at 65, most older people lead physically and socially active lives well into their eighties.

GROWTH AND DEVELOPMENT

Growth and development support a person in their progress throughout their life cycle (see the diagram opposite). However, as a person gets older, some aspects of growth and development slow down – parts of the body become worn out and this eventually leads to death.

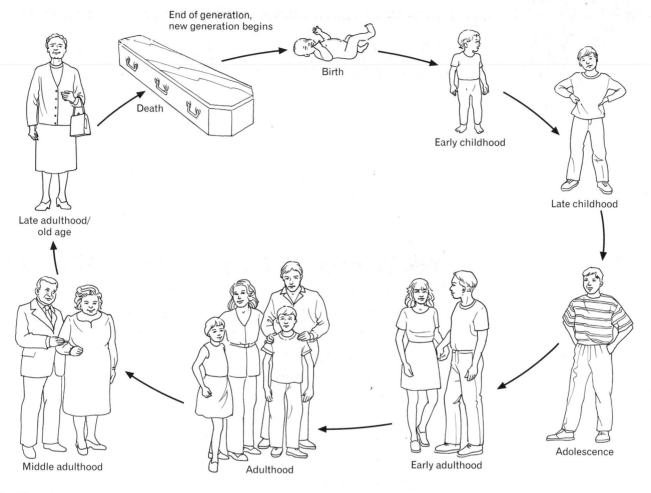

The life cycle

Physical effects of ageing

Ageing is a natural process which takes place in the different cells in the body. Each cell is programmed with information which is contained in a chemical called DNA (deoxyriboneucleic acid). The DNA instructs the cells to perform specific functions and to replace themselves when they are damaged or worn out. The cells make up a number of different tissues and organs which support the various systems in the body. These organs and systems depend on one another to function effectively and to remain in balance. The process which ensures this balanced internal environment is called homeostasis. The ageing body strives for homeostasis, and is usually successful in a stable, familar environment, but it cannot cope easily with stress, change or illness (Stoyle, 1991).

During the ageing process, however, cells do not always replace themselves – some cells deteriorate and die after suffering loss of function. There are several theories which provide reasons as to why this happens, and these are summarised in the diagram on page 148.

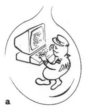

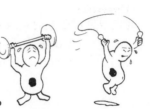

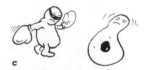

a

Genetic
Is life span programmed into the genes before birth?

b

Wear and tear
As cells wear out, are we less able to replace them?

c

Immune system
As older cells change are they attacked by the body's own immune system?

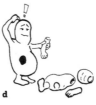

d

Error
As cells age do they make more mistakes in trying to replace themselves?

e

Cell death
Are the number of times the cell can reproduce itself programmed into the cell?

Theories of cellular ageing (Stoyle, 1991)

So what is the impact of cell change, cell death and the body's inability to replace every cell which becomes worn out? The overall effect is a decline in the function and efficiency of body systems, a slower metabolism and diminishing strength.

The physical aspects of ageing affect people in varying degrees. Some people age rapidly, while others maintain a high level of health and wellbeing. The most common physical effects are as follows (see also the diagram on page 152).

The digestive system

This includes organs such as the stomach, large and small intestines, liver, pancreas and rectum.

The movements in the digestive system are controlled by muscles. As part of the ageing process, these muscles become less efficient and this may cause problems with digestion of food, i.e. the food in the stomach is not reduced in size as effectively by the action of the stomach-wall muscles, so some of the food remains undigested. This can cause weight loss.

As the muscles of the gut wall weaken, it becomes more difficult to push the food along the alimentary canal so that the food stays in the gut or intestines for longer than it should. This results in constipation (see page 157).

Eyesight

Eyesight disorders include long-sighted vision and short-sighted vision. Other eye disorders which affect older people are cataracts and glaucoma (raised pressure inside the eye).

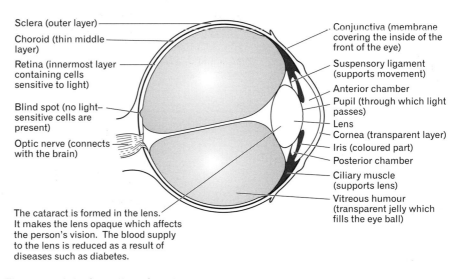

Sclera (outer layer)

Choroid (thin middle layer)

Retina (innermost layer containing cells sensitive to light)

Blind spot (no light–sensitive cells are present)

Optic nerve (connects with the brain)

Conjunctiva (membrane covering the inside of the front of the eye)

Suspensory ligament (supports movement)

Anterior chamber

Pupil (through which light passes)

Lens

Cornea (transparent layer)

Iris (coloured part)

Posterior chamber

Ciliary muscle (supports lens)

Vitreous humour (transparent jelly which fills the eye ball)

The cataract is formed in the lens. It makes the lens opaque which affects the person's vision. The blood supply to the lens is reduced as a result of diseases such as diabetes.

The eye and the formation of a cataract

Hair

Hair may lose its colour and turn grey. Grey hair is caused by the loss of the pigment which is found in each strand of hair. It is more common for men to lose hair, causing baldness.

The heart and the cardiovascular system

The function of the heart (see the diagram on page 150), which pumps blood around the body, becomes less efficient as a result of the ageing process. This means that less blood is circulated with each heart beat, and less blood reaches the body tissues. This can affect the general well-being of different parts of the body, such as the kidneys.

The reduced circulation of blood lowers the rate at which waste products are removed from the bloodstream. These waste products may build up and can affect the healthy functioning of the body.

Hearing

Ageing affects the ability to hear. This is first noticed by the number of high-pitched frequencies which are lost. Hearing what others are saying becomes more difficult. This may affect communication – an older person may appear to be ignoring others, but in fact may not be able to hear clearly what they are saying.

Heat regulating system

This monitors and regulates the amount of heat in the body. The ageing process affects the body in such a way that it becomes less efficient at maintaining itself at a constant temperature.

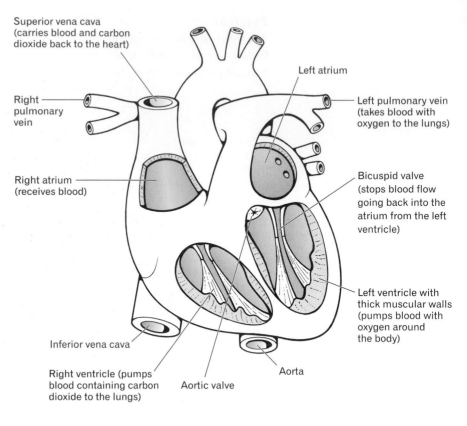

Superior vena cava
(carries blood and carbon
dioxide back to the heart)

Right
pulmonary
vein

Left atrium

Left pulmonary vein
(takes blood with
oxygen to the lungs)

Right atrium
(receives blood)

Bicuspid valve
(stops blood flow
going back into the
atrium from the left
ventricle)

Left ventricle with
thick muscular walls
(pumps blood with
oxygen around
the body)

Inferior vena cava

Aorta

Right ventricle (pumps
blood containing carbon
dioxide to the lungs)

Aortic valve

The mechanisms of the heart

In summer, an older person may quite happily wear a thick woolly cardigan to keep warm. In winter, older people become more vulnerable to the cold and their body temperature may drop, despite a number of layers of clothes. If their temperature drops too low, the person may suffer from **hypothermia**, which means that the body temperature is reduced and may not rise again without medical help.

Lungs and air passages
The lungs take in air from the atmosphere. They become less efficient during ageing.

An older person breathes in less air, which leads to breathlessness on exertion. Due to the reduced intake of air the lungs become less efficient. Once the air has been breathed in, the lungs remove oxygen to keep the body functioning. Ageing effects on the lungs may lead to complications as the heart has to work much harder to make up for the reduction of intake in oxygen from the lungs.

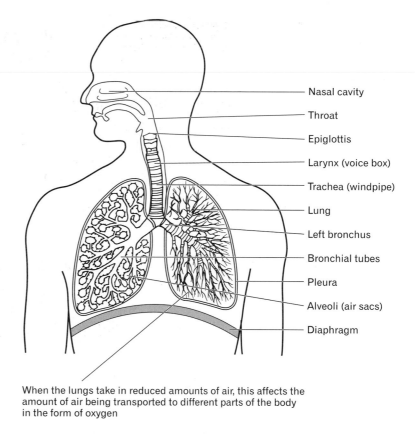

Nasal cavity

Throat

Epiglottis

Larynx (voice box)

Trachea (windpipe)

Lung

Left bronchus

Bronchial tubes

Pleura

Alveoli (air sacs)

Diaphragm

When the lungs take in reduced amounts of air, this affects the amount of air being transported to different parts of the body in the form of oxygen

The lungs and air passages

Metabolism

Chemical reactions in the body and the rate at which the body uses food and oxygen slow down during ageing. This may be due to various changes in the glands. The effects of ageing on metabolism may lead to tiredness, lethargy and lack of physical energy.

Reproductive system

Following the menopause, which marks the end of reproduction for women, the ovaries gradually become smaller and thicker. The secretions in the vagina are reduced which can make sexual intercourse painful. Men are still able to reproduce, but the number of sperm decreases and sexual arousal or erection may be slower.

Skeletal-muscular system

This consists of the joints, muscles and bone. During ageing, muscles gradually become less flexible, and bones may become more brittle and therefore likely to fracture.

151

Brittle bones are due to a reduction in the amount of calcium found in the bones. Calcium is a mineral essential for strong bones. Changes in the bones, and muscle degeneration, may cause people to lose height. Women in particular may be affected with brittle bones, because of the reduction of the hormone oestrogen during the menopause. This reduces the amount of calcium in the body and makes the person vulnerable to osteoporosis.

Skin

During ageing, skin loses its elasticity. This leads to wrinkles or lines which appear all over the body. The skin also tends to be drier, and patches of pigment may appear.

Urinary system

The urinary system includes the kidneys and the bladder. The general effects of ageing may lead to less efficient kidneys. The bladder capacity reduces due to muscle weakness, which leads to the need to pass urine more often.

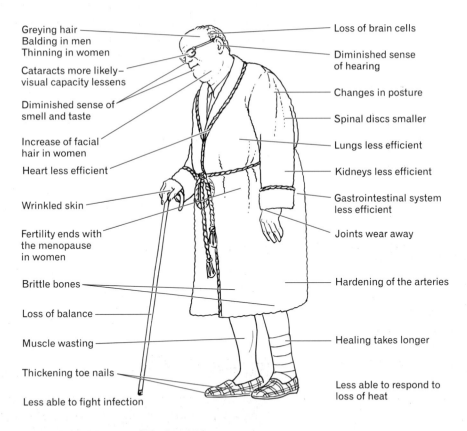

Physical effects of ageing (Stoyle, 1991)

Psychological and emotional effects of ageing

There are significant psychological changes which take place during the ageing process, which affect:

ACTIVITY

In groups:

a) Make a list of the methods you would use to support an older person who feels that their life has been useless and who is full of despair.

b) Decide whether you would use another older person who feels he has led a good life to support the despairing client.

- *the memory* – especially the short-term memory. This often results in older people becoming forgetful about the present, whilst still being able to recall their childhood and teenage years as if they were only yesterday. In some cases, this memory loss may become worse, and may lead to **confusion**. This is due to the fact that the brain, which is composed of millions of cells, helps the different parts body to function effectively. As part of the process of ageing the number of brain cells decreases.
- *the mind* – Changes in the mind vary from person to person. In most cases, older people tend to take longer to cope with problems and it may take them longer to learn something new. As a result, they prefer to 'stick to what they know' rather than try anything new. Sometimes, they may become stubborn and intolerant.

There are different psychological theories which consider the feelings, emotions and attitudes that relate to the process of ageing. One example of these theories was set out by the psychologist Erikson (1968). According to Erikson's table on page 68, older people are at *Stage 8 (Later life):* **Ego integrity** *versus despair.*

This is the final stage of the life cycle and explores the way in which older people review their lives in terms of how effective they feel that they have been during their lifetime. They may ask themselves questions such as 'Have I used my time wisely?' and 'Did I take all the opportunities which were available to me?'. Some may decide that they have had a productive life. This helps them to face their final years with a sense of satisfied resignation and enables them to maintain an interest in the world around them. On the other hand, an older person may reach a conclusion which leaves them with the feeling that they are useless. This can lead to despair. The role of the carer is particularly important with older people who have a despairing view of the remaining years of their lives.

Therefore, ego integrity relates to how the older person considers issues and events which have arisen in their lives. These include considering whether life has meaning or sense and should arrive at the conclusion that all life's experiences (positive and negative) have been valuable.

Social aspects of ageing

Ageing brings changes in social roles which include retirement from paid employment; this occurs regardless of the person's physical or mental health. This may cause them to feel useless, and to be unsure about how to pass all the extra time that they will have on their hands.

KEY POINT

Following retirement, older people still have a valuable role to play. Believing in this is an important factor in preserving their self-respect.

CASE STUDY

Maud

Maud is a retired teacher living in a flat in a large town. She taught in a local primary school for 25 years. She misses the contact with the other teachers and the children. She feels that her life is over. She has no children and her husband, who is also retired, has his own routine. She feels very lonely.

1 What advice would you give to Maud?

2 How would you support Maud in finding a way of overcoming her loneliness?

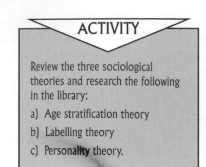

The sociological theories of ageing explore the different ways in which older people relate to the society in which they live. Some popular theories of ageing are:

- *Activity theory* – suggests that older people maintain an active role in society and view retirement as an opportunity to take up new interests and become involved in community action. Some elderly people may take up hobbies, such as swimming, painting, gardening or travel. Others may get actively involved with charity work, offering themselves as volunteers at the local shop

- *Continuity theory* – suggests that older people have individual personalities and that, as they grow older, their behaviour is more predictable. They tend to spend more time thinking and remembering the past rather than keeping up with their peers and maintaining a lifestyle

- *Disengagement theory* – suggests that older people disengage from the society in which they live, that they lose interest in the world around them as a way of preparing themselves for the end of their lives and for death.

Alongside these three theories, there are other social and economic factors which can affect the lives of older people. These factors include:

- *income and financial status* – the amount of money which older people have to live on. Do they have money which they have saved for old age? Are they receiving sufficient state pension? Are they finding it difficult to manage financially?

- *housing* – Where are older people living? Are they still in their own home? Have they moved into residential or sheltered housing?

- *culture* – the customs, beliefs, diet and religion which they have known throughout their lives. Are these being maintained?

- *social class* – the part of society with which they have formed associations through their occupation and employment, i.e working class, middle class and professional or upper class

- *health status* – the general health and well-being of an older person. Do they have a disability or chronic illness, such as arthritis?

- *lifestyle* – Do they maintain a lifestyle which involves a healthy diet, leisure pursuits, hobbies, holidays and travel?

BASIC NEEDS

Older people have various needs, which often relate to different aspects of the ageing process. The needs and rights of older people are summarised in Table 10.1.

Needs	Rights
Independence	● To be able to make decisions about their daily lives ● To live in a place of their own choice, preferably their own home whenever possible ● To receive support so that they can live as independently as possible
Affection	● To feel cared for and valued as individuals
Relationships	● To meet others of similar interests ● To build rapport and share experiences with others
Communication	● To be able to relate to others independent of disability or impairment ● To be given the appropriate equipment to promote communication, e.g. Bliss Boards, Braille books, etc.
Rest and sleep	● To be able to feel safe and protected and free from harm ● To live in a safe environment. Wherever possible, an older person's environment should be assessed with regard to their health and safety
Exercise and mobility	● To be able to take regular exercise ● To be encouraged to be as mobile as possible and, if appropriate, for suitable aids and equipment to be supplied
Dignity and self-respect	● To be respected for their individual beliefs ● To be encouraged to participate in activities which support their personal identity and promote positive self-esteem
Healthy diet	● To be supported with a diet which meets their needs. Support should be given if required with cooking, shopping or by the provision of meals-on-wheels
Routines, i.e. hygiene and toileting	● To be able to maintain the relevant routines necessary to support daily living ● To receive assistance if and when required
Stimulation	● To be able to continue with lifelong learning if they wish ● To meet with others for recreation such as reminiscence sessions and creative hobbies

Table 10.1 The needs and rights of older people

Social needs

The social needs of older people revolve around the long-term relationships which they have made during their lifetime. In some cases these relationships may diminish for a variety of reasons as people get older, such as retirement or when adult children move to a different part of the country. Therefore older people may experience:

- *loneliness* – a problem common in old age, not made any easier by the fact that elderly people have to face the fact that close family and friends will die. They may find it hard to make new friends as old ones die
- *changing roles* – such as parenting roles. They no longer have to care for their children. In fact, the roles are reversed and their children are often caring for them. Changing roles also include the loss of employment and, with this, the sense of identity that went with their job, such as being a farmer, nurse or teacher.

Physical needs

The physical needs of older people are mainly related to the process of ageing and any degeneration or disease which may occur. Examples of these are as follows.

Arthritis

Arthritis is inflammation of the joints. It can attack any age group but develops faster with ageing. There are two main types of arthritis:

- *osteo-arthritis*, which affects the larger joints, such as the knees and hips. It is the result of wear and tear on the joints, which is associated with ageing. It causes swelling and restriction of movement in the joints. The effects of osteo-arthritis can be reduced by taking regular exercise to strengthen the muscles supporting the joints and by following a weight-reducing diet
- *rheumatoid arthritis*, which includes symptoms such as fever, fatigue, loss of appetite and weight. Joints will become painful and swollen. These symptoms may be lessened through weight loss and regular exercise.

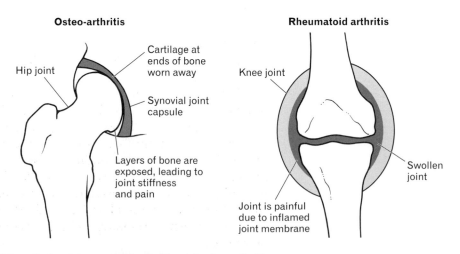

The effects of rheumatoid arthritis and osteo-arthritis

Constipation

This is a disorder where the bowel motions are hard, dry, and difficult to pass. It causes pain and discomfort and can result in haemorrhoids (piles) and other conditions. A healthy diet with plenty of fibre and fluids, and regular exercise, should help reduce constipation. Laxatives which are available from the chemist can also help.

Heart failure

Heart failure is a dysfunction in the heart when it is temporarily unable to pump enough blood around the body. Early symptoms are shortness of breath and fatigue, followed later by swollen ankles. Medical treatment is necessary to relieve the symptoms which may get worse if left unattended.

Hernias

A **hernia** occurs when a part of the body pushes through a weak point of the muscular wall. It occurs in different parts of the body. The most common hernia to affect older people is a rupture, when part of the bowel pushes through the abdominal wall. A hiatus hernia results from part of the stomach pushing through the muscular wall of the diaphragm. In severe cases, the hernia will need surgical treatment.

High blood pressure

This is when the pressure of blood pumping around the body is higher than it should be. The symptoms of **high blood pressure** include fatigue, breathlessness and chest pains, but some older people have no symptoms at all. In old age, higher blood pressure is quite normal, as it ensures that the blood is pushed up to the brain. If existing symptoms get worse, however, medical treatment is necessary.

Incontinence

This is when muscle control in the bladder and bowel has lost its elasticity. Bladder **incontinence** is more common than bowel incontinence. However, it may be due to an infection. If not, there is plenty of specialised equipment available.

Thrombosis

Thrombosis is when a blood clot develops in the arteries, caused by deposits in the arteries when they are not smooth and healthy. When thrombosis develops in the coronary artery (the artery supplying blood to the heart muscle), the person will suffer a heart attack – they will complain of pain in the chest which lasts for some time, and which may spread to the arms.

A clot of blood that passes to the brain will cause a stroke. The result of this is that a part of the brain will be temporarily or permanently out of action as it has been starved of vital blood supply. It is commonly thought that all strokes lead to paralysis and/or impairment of the senses. However, some strokes may be mild and are only detectable by changes in behaviour, such as difficulty in thinking, talking, walking or writing, or by a general lack of interest.

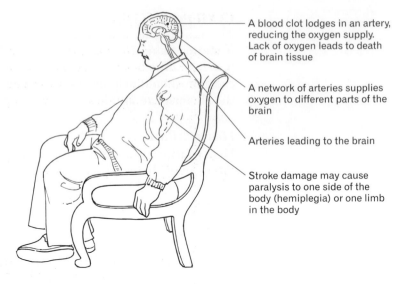

A blood clot lodges in an artery, reducing the oxygen supply. Lack of oxygen leads to death of brain tissue

A network of arteries supplies oxygen to different parts of the brain

Arteries leading to the brain

Stroke damage may cause paralysis to one side of the body (hemiplegia) or one limb in the body

What happens in a stroke

The result of a major stroke is that one side of the body is paralysed, and there may be speech loss. With physiotherapy and rehabilitation, stroke victims can regain a good deal of their independence.

To prevent strokes, older people should be encouraged to take plenty of exercise to keep the blood circulating, and to maintain a healthy diet.

Rheumatism

Rheumatism causes muscles or joints to stiffen and to ache. Rheumatism may be brought on by a number of factors, including cold weather, stress or poor posture. At the onset of pain, a mild pain-killer, such as aspirin, should help relieve the symptoms. The problem may increase with age, as the joints and muscles are then more prone to aches and pains.

Psychological and emotional needs

Due to the ageing process on different parts of the brain, some older people may suffer from:

- *confusion*, which is evident when an older person begins to lose touch with reality, and may imagine that they are being persecuted by others. Sometimes this may be due to dietary deficiency, glandular malfunction or infection

- *depression,* which is a psychological state when the older person feels very down and sad. The onset of depression may not be noticeable as it can be relatively mild. The older person may suffer from loss of appetite, lack of interest in their surroundings and disturbed sleep. Treatment is necessary if the depression worsens and the person begins to isolate themselves from others.

CARE ISSUES

The carer has a vital role to play in the lives of older people. It is important to recognise that older people are individuals, with many past experiences and memories that they may want to share. This is an integral part of their care.

Effective communication can support different tasks and activities with older clients.

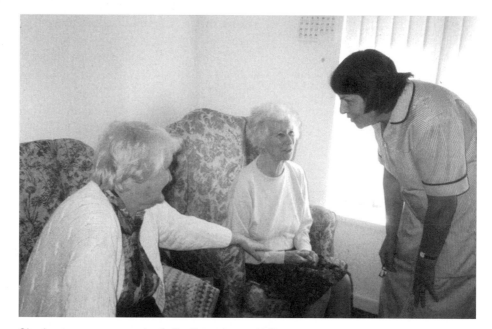

Sharing news: an example of effective communication

Emotional support

Giving emotional support as part of the caring process assists in promoting independence. Independence is important to the older person. The carer's role is to support that independence wherever possible. Keeping a client informed of all the issues which affect their lives is part of this.

Carers can involve clients by:

- *sharing information* – information which is relevant to older people relates to concerns about their health, their living conditions and their financial status. Keeping them regularly updated and making time to answer questions is part of this process. When clients are given regular information, they are more easily able to make decisions which may affect their future

- *supporting their rights and choices* – older clients have rights and choices and should be able to make decisions about the issues which affect them. The decision about their housing, their future care, where they will live and the carers who look after them are part of this. At the same time, their religious views, beliefs and culture should be considered as part of the individual rights and choices which support their needs.

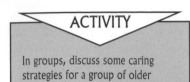

ACTIVITY

In groups, discuss some caring strategies for a group of older people in a day centre.

Older people can easily feel isolated and lonely. In most cases, every act of kindness is greatly appreciated. The caring attitude of the carer is discussed in Chapter 2 (page 12). It is important to:

- *show a caring attitude* – being supportive and sharing a genuine concern for clients should be an integral part of the care being given to older people. This can be difficult in cases where the client is confused or aggressive

- *show that the older person's contributions are valued* – listening to the person and making them feel that what they are saying is appreciated. Sometimes, the same story may be repeated on more than one occasion. Older people often have skills which can be shared with others, such as knitting and needlework. These skills can also be shared with a small group of children. Older people can work in a voluntary capacity in schools to listen to reading

- *retain the older person's dignity and self-respect* – older people should never be made to feel humiliated. They should be given respect and privacy, especially when they are being supported in hygiene and toileting tasks. Carers should always check that the client is dressed in clean and presentable clothes, i.e. appropriate day or night clothes.

Social relationships

Supporting relationships help the older person to keep up-to-date with the world around them. It assists their cognitive and intellectual development and helps to keep them alert.

Support communication and social networking

Having regular conversations is important to an older person who can become isolated and withdrawn from society and can feel that no one cares about them. Regular monitoring of older neighbours who live alone should be encouraged. Taking time to chat and to listen is an important requirement in caring for older people. Linking up with a local church or voluntary organisations is a way in which older people can be taken out to meet others.

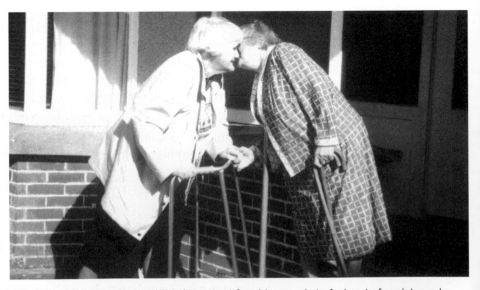

Meeting with others is great! It is important for older people to feel part of society and avoid a sense of isolation

Crisis contact

Older people ought to be able to contact others when they need help, for example, when they become unwell. Sheltered and residential care providers should have a alarm system to summon help. However, in the home, it can be different. Not all older people have telephones. Some older people do have a telephone alarm system which is activated by a small device which is worn around the client's neck. When they feel unwell, they press the button, which alerts the local ambulance station or emergency call centre.

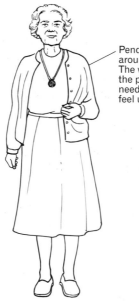

Pendant hangs around the neck. The wearer presses the pendant if they need help or feel unwell

Button which sounds when the pendant is pressed

Radio control–the person on duty calls the client to check on their condition. If there is no reply, help is sent

An emergency call system

Physical assistance

A most important requirement in working with older people is to ensure that they are able to be as independent as possible. This means that they should be encouraged to carry out tasks for themselves and, whenever necessary, equipment should be provided to support them.

Assessment of living skills

The necessary skills to maintain daily living are discussed in Chapter 5, pages 54–5. However, it is an important task for the carer to observe how an older client manages certain tasks. Giving support in using aids and equipment, showing the elderly person how to handle them, is essential.

Mobility

Whenever possible, clients should be encouraged to walk and exercise daily. There are various aids which can be used to support walking and mobility.

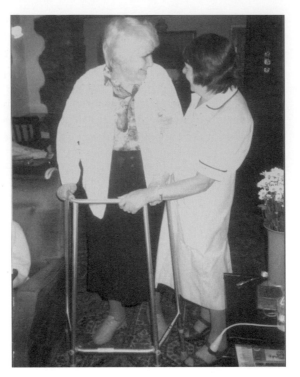

A walking frame is a useful aid to walking

Health and safety

The care setting or home should be safe. Carpets should be well tacked down and mats made firm. Handles should be easy to turn and all essential equipment should be kept within easy reach.

In residential care, health and safety requirements are covered by legislation such as the Health and Safety at Work Act 1974. Risk assessments should be regularly carried out with regard to handling and lifting clients (see Appendix 3).

Help with routines

Supporting older people with their daily routines is part of the role of the carer and care worker in different care settings. This will involve:

- *hygiene* – supporting clients with their washing and bathing is a regular task for carers working in residential care, for example, helping them in and out of the bath. In some cases, specialist equipment needs to be used. It is important to remember that carers should be specially trained to use equipment such as hoists
- *toileting* – supporting an older client with a toileting routine requires that they should be toileted on a regular basis. The carer should give the older person sufficient time to complete the task. The toilet door should be closed and the client's privacy maintained. Toileting is discussed further in Chapter 4, page 41
- *feeding* – checking that older people have a regular balanced diet, that they attend a local luncheon club, or receive meals-on-wheels. In a care setting,

older clients should be supported with their feeding if necessary. Wherever possible, relevant equipment should be purchased to support this. Feeding is discussed more fully in Chapter 4, page 38.

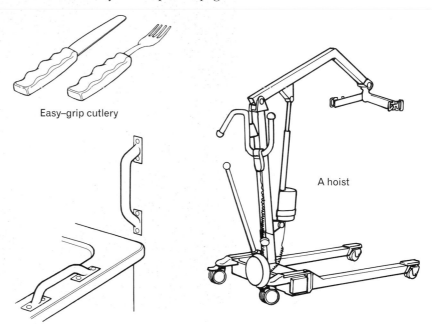

Easy–grip cutlery

A hoist

Rails in toilet, bath and shower

Aids to help with routines

KEY POINT

Carers should remember that older clients have the same needs as everyone else:

- They have a right to lead as independent a life as possible, surrounded by their own possessions and friends. This should be reviewed in terms of their long-term care.

- Once it has been accepted that an older person can no longer cope on their own, it is necessary to make a decision with regard to their future. It is important that this decision is shared by the older person concerned. There are many choices available, including sheltered accommodation and residential homes, but the decision depends on the needs of the individual concerned.

Financial support

Many older people find it difficult to manage on the money they have and find that they are unable to cope with an increasing cost of living.

The Benefits Agency is responsible for paying state pension to those of retirement age, and supplementary benefit to those whose incomes drop below a certain level. Additional income may come from private pension and insurance schemes, which the individual has contributed to during his or her working life.

Carers should support older clients by informing them of the various financial benefits which are available to them.

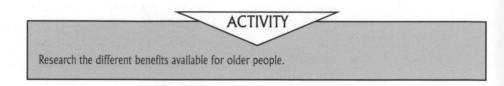

ACTIVITY

Research the different benefits available for older people.

LIFE EVENTS

Table 10.2 gives some examples of predictable events and unpredictable events which may occur in old age.

Predictable events	Unpredictable events
Ageing	Physical attack
Retirement	Elder abuse
Bereavement	Homelessness
Death	

Table 10.2 Predictable and unpredictable events in the lives of older people

Elder abuse

Elder abuse is a deliberate act to harm an older person. It can take the form of:

- *verbal abuse* – shouting and name calling
- *physical injury* – hitting them, handling them roughly, putting them in a hot bath or scalding them
- *neglect* – leaving them to sit in soiled and dirty clothes
- *emotional abuse* – stripping them naked in front of others.

Whenever abuse to an older person is suspected, it should be reported to the manager of the care setting. However, older people may not want to complain, because they fear the situation will only get worse.

Death and bereavement

The most predictable event for an older person is death, both the death of others and, ultimately, their own death, possibly after long illness. They will encounter the loss of many of their friends and family. Bereavement is something which older people experience more than other age groups. The grief process is part of bereavement. Table 10.3 outlines the process of grief and methods of support.

Grief	Stages	Determinants of grief	Coping mechanisms	Method of support
• Loss of a loved one which is a major stress in the life of an individual • Reaction to loss of a relationship, object, status, social role, employment	• Numbness – a psychological and physical barrier which blocks out pain • Searching and pining – lack of concentration, thinks only of the person and their death • Depression – reaction to death, realises and is forced to accept the person is not coming back • Recovery – begins to pick up threads of life again	These affect the outcomes of the grieving process. They can predict difficulties which occur as the person works through grief process: • Mode of death – how the death occurred • Nature of the attachment – the strength of the relationship • Who was the person? What was the contact with the person? • Historical antecedents – any previous experience of bereavement • Personality variables – personality characteristics or traits • Social variables – does the death isolate the client or is it an opportunity to join groups?	• Philosophical – everyone has to die some time • Denial – the person has not died. It can't be true • Anger – anger is directed at another person or object, e.g. the bereaved may complain about hospitals/ doctors, etc. • Looking forward and finding ways to cope with loss	• Building supportive relationships • Listening to the client talk about the loss and letting them remember • Offering advice and information with regard to different groups, e.g. CRUSE

Table 10.3 The process of grief, coping mechanisms and methods of support (based on Parkes, 1975)

SOURCES OF SUPPORT

Older people need individual support in a number of areas.

KEY POINT

Caring for older people and supporting their independence can be a satisfying and positive experience. They are sources of interesting information who should be appreciated and not discarded.

Professional support

Older people receive health support through their local GP surgery and hospital. There are a range of professionals who support older people, including:

- GP and Primary Health Care team
- chiropodist – to care for their feet
- physiotherapist – to support their mobility
- occupational therapist – to support their independence in the home.

Organisations which support older people

Age Concern, Astral House, 1268 London Road, London SW16 4ER

Alzheimer's Disease Society, 2nd Floor, Gordon House, 10 Greencoat Place, London SW1P 1PH

Arthritis and Rheumatism Council, Copeman House, St Mary's Court, St Mary's Gate, Chesterfield, Derbyshire S41 7TD

Association for Residential Care, ARC House, Marsden, Chesterfield, Derbyshire S40 1LR

Centre for Policy on Ageing, 25–31 Ironmonger Row, London EC1V 3QP

Cruse Bereavement Care, Cruse House, 126 Sheen Road, Richmond, Surrey TW9 1UR

Disabled Living Foundation, 380–384 Harrow Road, London W9 2HU

Help the Aged, St James Walk, London EC1R OBE

National Osteoporosis Society, PO Box 10, Radstock, Bath, Avon

Research Institute in Care of the Elderly, St Martin's Hospital, Bath, Avon BA2 5RP

Research into Ageing – Improving the Quality of Life, Baird House, 15–17 St Cross Street, London EC1N 3UN

Stroke Association, CHSA House, Whitecross Street, London WC1Y 8JJ

Victim Support, Cramner House, 39 Brixton Road, London SW9

WRVS Trust, 234–244 Stockwell Road, London SW9 9SP

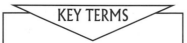

KEY TERMS

You need to know the meaning of the following words and phrases. Go back through to the chapter to make sure that you understand them.

Activity theory
arthritis
confusion
Continuity theory
depression
Disengagement Theory
ego integrity
elder abuse
heart failure
hernia
high blood pressure
hypothermia
incontinence
rheumatism
thrombosis

Glossary

Activity theory a way of explaining how people react to old age. It suggests that older people can maintain an active role in society and can view retirement as an opportunity to take up new interests and become involved in community action

acute health care services medical and surgical treatments and follow-up care, for example emergency health services, district general hospitals, nursing homes

adolescence the life stage that begins at puberty and ends with the onset of adulthood

adulthood the longest period of the lifespan; it covers a range of changes over approximately 47 years; it begins at 18 when the young person becomes eligible to vote, and extends to 65 years of age and beyond

advocate a person who represents the interests of another person, speaking on their behalf where they are unable, for whatever reason, to speak for themselves

anti-discriminatory care care that seeks to challenge and reduce individual and institutional discrimination against clients on grounds of, for example, race, gender, disability, social class, age and sexual orientation

arthritis a condition caused by inflammation of the joints resulting in swelling, pain and restriction of movement

assessment the process of identifying the needs of an individual client

associative play occurs when a child is 3+ years old and involves play with other children in small groups

autonomy another word for self-government or self-determination. Care practice should promote clients' autonomy by giving choices, allowing clients to make their own decisions wherever possible and by minimising control over their lives

barriers to communication behaviours which can hinder effective communication between individuals

behaviour a child's or an individual's conduct, acceptable and unacceptable ways of carrying out actions and speaking to others

birth injuries injuries which occur during the delivery of a baby and may result in temporary or permanent damage to the bones, muscles, nerves and skin. Bones can fracture, nerves can be stretched and damaged, particularly those that supply the neck

bonding the forming of a close relationship between a baby and primary care-givers

burn-out the outcome of experiencing very high **stress** levels at work. A person who is 'burnt out' tends to have continuous feelings of exhaustion, tension and negative attitudes to work

care plan   a document that outlines the care objectives and the strategies chosen for meeting them

care planning   the process of **assessment** of a client's needs and planning the care, treatment or therapy between professional carers and their clients. The resulting plan of care is called the **care plan**

care relationship the relationship which is built up between a carer or care worker and a client

Care Value Base   the key values of the caring profession, which ensure clients are treated equally and fairly in terms of their right to support through effective communication: **confidentiality** and **privacy**; having individual's choices respected; having personal beliefs acknowledged and acted upon; receiving **anti-discriminatory care**

challenging behaviour   demanding or threatening behaviour, outbursts of verbal abuse and stubbornness which can be accompanied by aggressive and violent actions

child abuse   harm to a child which may be physical, sexual, emotional, or caused by neglect

child health surveillance   the observation and monitoring of a child's pattern of growth and development during the first year of life. Health visitors carry out child health surveillance through the use of various developmental and screening tests

confidentiality   the principle of protecting the personal and health information of clients receiving care and only discussing this with, or disclosing it to, other members of a care team if necessary, or to others only with the client's permission

confusion   when an older person begins to lose touch with reality, and may imagine that they are being persecuted by others. Sometimes this may be due to dietary deficiency, glandular malfunction or infection

constructive play   play that involves putting objects, such as bricks, together in a purposeful way

continuing care services   continuous care services, which are provided to meet the ongoing, different health and social care needs of individuals with chronic (long-term) conditions, for example care services for older people, home-help services

Continuity theory   a way of explaining how older people deal with old age. It is argued that older people have individual personalities but that, as they grow older, their behaviour is more predictable. They tend to spend more time thinking and remembering the past rather than keeping up with their peers and maintaining a lifestyle

co-operative play   demonstrated by children aged 3+ who play and learn together by giving each other roles and responsibilities within a group

creative play   involves the use of different materials, such as paint, water and sand, in imaginative activities

cultural needs the need for one's individual cultural expectations and realities to be respected; see **culture**

culture the different beliefs, values and customs that define an individual's lifestyle and pattern of daily living

day care care carried out in a day centre or day hospital.

depression a psychological state when an older person feels very down and sad; the onset may not be noticeable as it can be relatively mild. The older person may suffer from loss of appetite, lack of interest in their surroundings and disturbed sleep. Treatment is necessary if the depression worsens and the older person begins to isolate themselves from others

discrimination unfair treatment of a person or group of people because of prejudice, intolerance and ignorance; can be based on race (racism), gender (sexism), age (ageism), disability, sexuality, religion, health status, cognitive ability or political persuasion; can be direct (overt) or indirect (covert)

Disengagement theory the idea that older people gradually disengage from society, losing interest in the world around them, as a way of preparing themselves for death

divorce legal and permanent separation; the end of a marriage

domestic violence abuse which occurs within a partnership or family; involves power and control by one person within the relationship; one partner uses physical, emotional, economic, sexual or psychological means to exercise control over the other

domiciliary care care carried out in a client or service user's own home

drug misuse the use of substances for non-medical/non-therapeutic purposes; the act of taking illegal drugs such as heroin, marijuana, cocaine, amphetamines and LSD is a form of drug misuse; the inappropriate use of prescription drugs and solvents

eating disorder conditions such as anorexia nervosa and bulimia nervosa which involve the sufferer inappropriately restricting and controlling their food intake to reduce their weight and cope with psychological problems relating to physical appearance and body shape

ego integrity a theory determined by Erikson, 1968, it explains how the older person considers issues and events which have arisen in their lives, including whether life has meaning or sense, and should arrive at the conclusion that all life's experiences (positive and negative) have been valuable.

elder abuse a deliberate act to harm an older person. It can be verbal, physical, neglect or emotional

emotional needs the need to feel accepted, secure and positive about yourself

empathy the ability to appreciate another person's feelings, to see the situation from the other person's point of view

empower to enable a client or service user to gain and maintain control over their life

failure to thrive when a baby does not appear to grow at the expected rate. Reasons for this condition may include a feeding disorder, an allergy to milk, difficulty in absorbing food, being prone to infection, little or no stimulation in the home environment

fine motor skills   the small body movements needed to manipulate and control movement and physical activity. Fine motor skills are needed to hold and examine an object in the hand

five Cs of caring   compassion, conscience, commitment, confidence, competence (Roach, 1987)

formal care care provided by professional, employed carers who look after and support individuals in formal care settings, for example, registered general nurses, health care assistants, district nurses, health visitors

generativity   the adult is concerned for others and life beyond the immediate family. They may be involved with community and voluntary work

gross motor skills   the large body movements that enable a person to be physically active and well co-ordinated. Running and jumping involve gross motor skills

healthy diet   a diet which provides sufficient energy (calories) to enable the person to maintain normal body weight. The diet should include daily amounts of fats, proteins, carbohydrates, vitamins, minerals, fibre, water, and trace elements in the correct balance

heart failure   a dysfunction of the heart where the ability to pump blood around the body is reduced or impaired

hernia   when an organ or tissue pushes through a weak point of the muscular wall and moves out of the body cavity in which it normally lies

high blood pressure   when the pressure of blood pumping around the body is higher than it should be; symptoms include fatigue, breathlessness and chest pains, but some older people have no symptoms at all

holistic care   an approach to the caring process which assesses and meets *all the different needs* of an individual. The care recognises the requirements of the *whole person* – their **physical needs**, **intellectual and cognitive needs**, **social needs**, **emotional needs**, **spiritual needs** and **cultural needs**

hospital care care involving complex medical or surgical interventions or an emergency admission

hypothermia   when the body temperature drops too low; it may not rise again without medical help

immunisation   administering vaccines to produce artificial immunity, to protect people against infectious diseases such as polio. Many immunisation programmes are targeted at babies and children

incontinence   involuntary passage of urine or faeces from the bladder or bowel as a result of lost muscle control, leakage or stress reaction

infertility   the inability of a woman to conceive or a man to induce conception

informal care care provided by relatives, friends, volunteers or neighbours who give support and care for an individual, usually in that person's home, without pay

inherited disease   a condition that is passed from one generation of a family to another through genetic transfer/chromosomes.

intellectual and cognitive needs   the need for learning and education

labelling   the attribution of a quality or feature, usually negative, to an individual or group of people so that they come to be defined by it. For example, people who experience mental illness are often labelled as 'dangerous' and 'unpredictable' when this is not usually true

lifelong learning   a process whereby a person's educational needs can be met in the adult years

living skills   skills that enable a person to carry out their daily activities in order to maintain their lifestyle. Food preparation might be seen as an essential living skill

make-believe play   involves role play and imaginative play. Children will imitate adult actions and will enjoy dressing up and playing games like 'hospitals'

menopause   affects women between their late thirties and early fifties; it is the process that ends with the ceasing of the reproductive function; the ovaries reduce the production of the hormone oestrogen and menstruation becomes irregular and eventually ceases. Some women can suffer side effects such as headaches, tension, mood swings, hot flushes and osteoporosis

National Curriculum   the curriculum which must be taught to all children of statutory school age (i.e. 5–16 years) in the UK

non-verbal communication   body language (gestures and postures), facial expression, use of personal space, body contact

parallel play   demonstrated by children aged 2–3 years old who enjoy playing independently alongside each other

peer group   a group of people who are of the same age or who share particular interests

phenylketonuria (PKU)   an inherited disorder caused by the presence of excess phenylalanine in the blood. It results in damage to the nervous system and mental retardation. All new-born babies are screened for PKU using the Guthrie test and can be successfully treated if the disorder is noticed early enough

physical needs   the need to maintain the functioning of the body by keeping warm, healthy, safe, clean, fit

prejudice   prejudgement of person or group of people based on stereotyped attitudes; can result in **discrimination**

primary care 'front-line', community-based, non-hospital services such as school health services, home nursing services and GP services

primary sexual characteristics   the physical features in the body that are present from birth which determine whether an individual is male or female– in boys they are the penis and testes and in girls the vagina and ovaries

priority services emergency or immediate care services, for example, ambulance services

privacy   in care settings, the right of an individual to their own personal space

puberty the period during which **secondary sexual characteristics** develop and the reproductive organs become functional, enabling an individual to reproduce – in girls, puberty usually starts between the ages of 10 and 13, while in boys it starts a little later, between 12 and 14 years

residential care care provided in settings where clients live all the time, such as residential homes, nursing homes and hostels

rheumatism a condition which causes muscles or joints to stiffen and ache

secondary care 'second line' services, usually hospital-based care such as acute services provided through a district general hospital

secondary sexual characteristics appear during **puberty** when the primary reproductive organs in males and females grow and mature – in boys they include the growth of facial and pubic hair and 'breaking' of the voice; in girls they include the growth of pubic hair and development of the breasts

self-awareness both the process and the outcome of getting to know your feelings, attitudes and values, and the effect that you have on others

self-concept the way in which a person views and evaluates themself, often in comparison to other people

self-help skills skills which are necessary to carry out different tasks and activities to maintain daily living and independence; see also **living skills**

sensory impairment a disability that affects sight, hearing, smell, taste or touch

sexually-transmitted diseases (STDs) infections, such as syphilis and gonorrhoea, that result from unprotected sexual intercourse with an infected partner

social care services care services which support the physical, intellectual, emotional, social and cultural needs of the individual, for example, residential care, day care

social needs the need to meet others, to have friends

social role a position in society which requires a person to act in particular ways (mother, nurse, wife, sister). People often perceive themselves in terms of the social roles that they undertake

socialisation the process whereby people are taught the 'correct' ways to behave in a society; they learn attitudes, values and behaviours from close family members at first and later from peers, teachers and work colleagues

solitary play demonstrated by children up to the age of 2 who will play alone, although they may prefer to have a parent present in the background

special need any condition that may affect an individual's health or well-being

spiritual needs the need to fulfil a belief or realise self-fulfilment through one means or another; the need to have one's religious beliefs respected

stagnation the adult becomes increasingly concerned with themselves and their lifestyle. They are constantly pre-occupied with their personal needs and they can become fixed in their views and attitudes

stereotype a fixed view a person has about another person or group of people, linked to certain (often inaccurate) characteristics of individuals; can result in **prejudice** and **discrimination**

stress   unwelcome pressure and the resultant feeling of being unable to cope with demands on one's time and abilities

stress management   strategies to manage stress through diet, talking, exercise or time off

tertiary care 'third line' care in specialist institutions, such as the Royal Marsden Hospital, which specialises in cancer care

thrombosis   when a blood clot develops in the arteries, caused by deposits in the arteries which are not smooth and healthy. In the coronary artery, the result is a heart attack; in the brain it will cause a stroke

weaning   the gradual introduction of solid food into a baby's diet

Appendices

Code of Professional Conduct for Nurses, Midwives and Health Visitors

This code of practice was drawn up by the UKCC (the United Kingdom Central Council for Nursing, Midwifery and Health Visiting), a professional body for registered nurses, midwives or health visitors who should act, at all times, in such a manner as to:

- safeguard and promote the interests of individual patients and clients
- serve the interests of society
- justify public trust and confidence and
- uphold and enhance the good standing and reputation of the professions.

The Code continues:
As a registered nurse, midwife or health visitor, you are personally accountable for your practice and, in the exercise of your professional accountability, must:

- act always in such a manner as to promote and safeguard the interests and well-being of patients and clients
- ensure that no action or omission on your part, or within their sphere of responsibility, is detrimental to the interests, condition or safety of patients and clients
- maintain and improve your professional knowledge and competence
- acknowledge any limitations in your knowledge and competence and decline any duties or responsibilities unless able to perform them in a safe and skilled manner
- work in an open and co-operative manner with patients, clients and their families, foster their independence and recognise and respect their involvement in the planning and delivery of care
- work in an collaborative and co-operative manner with health-care professionals and others involved in providing care, and recognise and respect their particular contributions within the care team
- recognise and respect the uniqueness and dignity of each patient and client, and respond to their need for care, irrespective of their ethnic origin, religious beliefs, personal attributes, the nature of their health problems or any other factor
- report to an appropriate person or authority, at the earliest possible time, any conscientious objection which may be relevant to your professional practice

- avoid any abuse of your privileged relationship with patients and clients and of the privileged access allowed to their person, property, residence or workplace

- protect all confidential information concerning patients and clients obtained in the course of professional practice and make disclosures only with consent, where required by the order of a court or where you can justify disclosure in the wider public interest

- report to an appropriate person or authority, having regard to the physical, psychological and social effects on patients and clients, any circumstances in the environment of care which could jeopardise standards of practice

- report to an appropriate person or authority any circumstances in which safe and appropriate care for patients and clients cannot be provided

- report to an appropriate person where it appears that the health or safety of colleagues is at risk, as such circumstances may compromise standards of practice and care

- assist professional colleagues, in the context of your own knowledge, experience and sphere of responsibility, to develop their professional competence, and assist others in the care team, including informal carers, to contribute safely and to a degree appropriate to their roles

- refuse any gift, favour or hospitality from patients or clients currently in your care which might be interpreted as seeking to exert influence to obtain preferential consideration and

- ensure that your registration status is not used in the promotion of commercial products or services, declare any financial or other interests in relevant organisations providing such goods or services and ensure that your professional judgement is not influenced by any commercial considerations.

This Code of Professional Conduct for the Nurse, Midwife and Health Visitor is issued to all registered nurses, midwives and health visitors by the United Kingdom Central Council for Nursing, Midwifery and Health Visiting. The Council is the regulatory body responsible for the standards of these professions and it requires members of the professions to practise and conduct themselves within the standards and framework provided by the Code (UKCC, 1992, reproduced by permission).

APPENDIX 1B

Code of Professional Practice for Social Workers

This material first appeared in the British Association of Social Workers *Code of Ethics*, published and reproduced by kind permission of the British Association of Social Workers.

Each qualified social worker is required to act in a way that demonstrates the following:

- positively using knowledge, skills and experience for the benefit of all sections of the community and individuals

- respecting clients as individuals and safeguarding their dignity and rights

- ensuring that there is no prejudice which is evident to others, on grounds of origin, race, status, sex, sexual orientation, age, disability, beliefs or contribution to society
- empowering clients and encouraging their participation in decisions and defining services
- sustaining concern for clients even when they are unable to help them or where self-protection is necessary
- making sure that professional responsibility takes precedence over personal interest
- being responsible for standards of service and for continuing education and training
- collaborating with others in the interests of clients
- ensuring clarity in public as to whether acting in a personal or organisational capacity
- promoting appropriate ethnic and cultural diversity of services
- ensuring confidentiality of information and divulging only by consent or exceptionally in the event of serious danger
- pursuing conditions of employment which enable these obligations to be respected (British Association of Social Workers, 1992).

APPENDIX 2

Care: principles of good practice

The agreed principles which underpin the National Occupational Standards in health and social care are:

- balancing people's rights with their responsibilities to others and to wider society and challenging those who affect the rights of others
- promoting the values of equality and diversity, acknowledging the personal beliefs and preferences of others and promoting anti-discriminatory practice
- maintaining the confidentiality of information, provided that this does not place others at risk
- recognising the effect of the wider social, political and economic context on health and social well-being and on people's development
- enabling people to develop to their full potential, to be as autonomous and self-managing as possible and to have a voice and be heard
- recognising and promoting health and social well-being as a positive concept
- balancing the needs of clients who use services with the resources available and exercising financial probity
- developing effective relationships with people and maintaining the integrity of these relationships through setting appropriate role boundaries
- developing oneself and one's own practice to improve the quality of services offered
- working within statutory and organisational frameworks (Care Sector Consortium, 1998).

APPENDIX 3

Moving and handling: manual techniques for moving people

Moving and handling are techniques taught by a recognised trainer identifying the weight guidelines which are described in the Health and Safety Executive booklet (*Guidance on the Regulations: Manual handling of loads*).

Moving clients involves principles of handling such as:

- before moving anything, thinking and planning ahead
- arranging the room and ensuring that the appropriate equipment has space to function
- ensuring that the weight and load is appropriate for the people involved in the technique
- assessment prior to the moving and handling will review the client's ability to move, the carer's ability to move and handle and the way in which the task will be carried out in the care environment
- all carers should be trained in the different techniques in lifting and handling and the use of handling equipment.

The choice of moving and handling technique will often depend on the:

- client and the way in which they are able to move for themselves
- weight and size of the client
- other people involved in the exercise.

Equipment used in lifting and handling includes:

- different hoists
- patient handling slings
- transfer boards
- turntables
- hand blocks.

Moving and handling techniques should ensure that the health and well-being of both client and carer are taken into account. There have been many cases where carers have injured their backs through handling patients without proper training.

Health and Safety at Work Act 1974

Under this Act, everyone has a legal duty to uphold certain standards of health, safety and welfare. Employers must ensure the health, safety and welfare of their employees, so far as is reasonably practicable. This means providing:

- relevant information, instruction training and supervision
- safe equipment and working methods (including property maintenance)
- safe arrangements for the use, handling, storage and transport of all articles and substances
- safe working environment

- a written health and safety policy
- a safety committee when required
- protective clothing, equipment and safety devices as necessary, at no charge.

Employees also have their own responsibilities under the Act. Employees must:

- take reasonable care for the health and safety of themselves and others who may be affected by their acts or omissions
- co-operate with their employer to enable him/her to comply with any duty or requirement imposed on him/her
- not intentionally or recklessly interfere with or misuse anything provided by law for their health, safety or welfare.

Employees should also take note of safety rules provided for their protection. They should:

- not attempt to carry out any work unless they have been specifically trained to do so, and are confident of their ability
- report unsafe equipment or situations
- report all accidents at work
- study the safety policy and procedures provided for them and their part in complying with them.

Health and Safety at Work Regulations 1992

These are in response to six new EC Directives and form part of the Health and Safety at Work Act. EC Directive 90.269/EEC 'Manual Handling of Loads' is part of these regulations. This Directive is important for any employer and employee involved in the manual handling of loads during the course of their work.

The Directive lays down minimum Health and Safety requirements for the manual handling of loads where there is a risk, particularly of back injury, to workers.

Manual handling is defined by the Directive as supporting a load by one or more workers including:

- lifting
- putting down
- pushing
- pulling
- carrying a load
- moving a load.

General measures to be taken:

- **Avoid** hazardous manual handling so far as is reasonably practical.
- **Assess** – make a suitable and sufficient assessment of any hazardous manual handling operation that cannot be avoided.
- **Reduce risk**, i.e. **use mechanical devices**.

Duties of employers:

- Avoid manual handling.
  - Use mechanical aids.
  - Eliminate task.
- Assess all moving and handling tasks.
  - Who does it?
  - Assess:
    task
    load
    environment
    individual
- Reduce the risk and assess
  - equipment
  - environment (space)
  - load
  - repetition
  - training
  - weight guidelines.

Duties of employees:

- Follow approved systems.
- Make use of equipment.
- Co-operate with employers.

APPENDIX 4

First aid

First aid is the immediate assistance or treatment given to someone injured or suddenly taken ill before the arrival of an ambulance, doctor or other appropriately qualified person. The person offering this help to a casualty must act calmly and with confidence and, above all, must be willing to offer assistance whenever the need arises. However, first aid is a skill based on knowledge, training and experience. The term 'first aider' is usually applied to someone who has completed a theoretical and practical instruction course and passed the professionally supervised examination. The standard First Aid Certificate, which is awarded by the St John Ambulance, St Andrew's Ambulance and the British Red Cross, is proof of all-round competence.

The aims of first aid

- To preserve life
- To limit worsening of the condition
- To promote recovery

The responsibilities of first aiders

- To assess a situation quickly and safely and to summon appropriate help
- To protect casualties and others at the scene from possible danger

- To identify, as far as possible, the injury or nature of the illness affecting the casualty

- To give each casualty early and appropriate treatment, dealing with the most serious conditions first

- To arrange for a casualty's removal to hospital into the care of a doctor or to his or her home

- To remain with a casualty until appropriate care is available

- To report your observations to those taking over care of the casualty and to give further assistance if required

First aid regulations and legislation

First aid may be practised in any situation where accidents or illnesses have occurred. In many instances, the first person on the scene is a volunteer who wants to help rather than someone who is medically trained. That person may or may not have a knowledge of first aid procedures and treatments. It is important to remember that the Health and Safety and First Aid Regulations 1981 place a general duty on employers to make first aid provision for employees in case of injury or illness in the workplace.

In the different aspects of caring, it is important for carers to learn what to do in an emergency; the St John Ambulance offer a number of steps to enable a carer to take action:

1 Assess the situation – are there risks to you or to the casualty?
2 Assess the casualty – is the casualty visibly conscious, if he has collapsed does he respond to shaking of the shoulders?
3 Assess the condition
4 Move on to resuscitation if breathing is absent – open the airway, check the breathing
5 Breathe for the casualty
6 Assess the circulation
7 Commence cardio-pulmonary resuscitation (CPR).

These extracts have been taken from the *First Aid Manual* which is authorised by the St John Ambulance, St Andrew's Ambulance Association and the British Red Cross (1997). Wherever possible, carers should learn an emergency procedure, especially if they are working with clients in their own homes. Obviously legislation covers the first aid procedures in the workplace. However, there are still the unpredictable accidents which happen in the street and which are, in some cases, life-threatening. The appropriate first aid treatment given in these situations is often life-saving prior to the arrival of the Ambulance Service.

References

Adams, R. (1994) *Skilled Work with People*, London: Collins Educational

Barnes, P. (1998) *Personal, Social and Emotional Development of Children*, Open University/Blackwell

Beaver, M., Brewster, J., Jones, P., Keene, A., Neaum, S. and Tallack, J. (1999) *Babies and Young Children, Book 1: Early Years Development*, 2nd edition, Cheltenham: Stanley Thornes

Beaver, M., Brewster, J., Jones, P., Keene, A., Neaum, S. and Tallack, J. (1999) *Babies and Young Children, Book 2: Early Years Care and Education*, 2nd edition, Cheltenham: Stanley Thornes

Beaver, M. Brewster, J. and Keene, A. (1997) *Child Care and Education*, Cheltenham: Stanley Thornes

Biesteck, F.P. (1992) *The Casework Relationship*, London: Routledge

Bowlby, J. (1951) *Maternal Care and Mental Health*, Geneva: World Health Organisation

Brain, J. and Martin, M.D. (1995) *Child Care and Health*, Cheltenham: Stanley Thornes

British Association of Social Workers (1992) *Code of Professional Practice for Social Workers*, British Association of Social Workers

Brown, H. and Basset, T. (1996) *New Lifestyles for Carers*, Pavilion Publishing

Burnard, P. (1992) *Communication Skills Guide for Health Care Workers*, London: Edward Arnold

Care Sector Consortium (1998) *Local Government Management Board*, London: The Stationery Office

Carers Recognition and Services Act (1995) London: The Stationery Office

Clarke, L., Rowell, K. and White, M. (1992) *A First Course in Caring*, Cheltenham: Stanley Thornes

Clarke, L., Sachs, B. and Ford, S. (1995) *GNVQ Advanced Health and Social Care*, 2nd edition, Cheltenham: Stanley Thornes

Clarke, L., Sachs, B. and Waltham, P. (1994) *GNVQ Advanced Health and Social Care*, Cheltenham: Stanley Thornes

Counsel & Care (1990) *Not only Bingo*, London: Counsel & Care

Counsel & Care (1995) *Leisure, Later Life and Homes*, London: Counsel & Care

Dare, A. and O'Donovan, M. (1998) *Working With Babies*, 2nd edition, Cheltenham: Stanley Thornes

Erikson, E. (1963) *Childhood and Society,* Norton

First Aid Manual (1997) Dorling Kindersley

Health & Safety At Work Act (1974) London: The Stationery Office

Holmes, T.H. and Rahe, R.H. (1967) 'The social readjustment rating scale', *Journal of Psychosomatic Research*, 11, 213–1218

Home From Home (1992) London: The Stationery Office

King's Fund (1995) *10 Point Plan*, Carers' National Association

Maslow, A. (1970) *Motivation and Personality*, New York: Harper Row

Miller, J. (1996) *Social Care Practice*, Hodder & Stoughton

Modell, J. and Goodman, M. (1990) 'Historical perspectives', in Feldman, S.S. and Elliott, G.R. (eds) *At the Threshold: The Developing Adolescent*, Cambridge, Mass: Harvard University Press

Morrison, P. and Burnard, P. (1992) *Caring and Communicating*, Macmillan Nursing Books

Moonie, N., Ixer, G., Makepeace, K. and Balkissoon, I., (1995) *Human Behaviour in a Caring Context*, Cheltenham: Stanley Thornes

NHS and Community Care Act (1995) London: The Stationery Office

Nouwen, H.J., McNeil and Morrison, D.A. (1982) *Compassion*, Harlow: Longman

Oxford Dictionary of Current English (1985) Oxford: Oxford University Press

Parker, G and Lawton. D. (1994) *Different Types of Care, Different Types of Carer: Evidence from the General Household Survey*, London: The Stationery Office

Parkes, C. (1975) *Bereavement: Study in Grief in Adult Life*, Harmondsworth: Penguin

Platt Report (1959) *The Welfare of Children in Hospital*, London: HMSO

Roach, Simone M. (1987) *The Human Act of Caring*, Ottawa: Canadian Hospital Association

Rope, N., Logan, W. and Tierney, A. (1990) *The Elements of Nursing*, Churchill Livingstone

Stoyle, J (1991) *Caring for Older People*, Cheltenham: Stanley Thornes

Tackling Drugs Together – To Build A Better Britain (1998) London: The Stationery Office

Thomson, H., Holden, C., Hutt, G., Meggitt, C., Manual, J. and Collard, D. (1995) *Health and Social Care*, 2nd edition, Hodder & Stoughton

Tschudin, V. (1995) *Ethics in Nursing*, Butterworth-Heinemann

UKCC (1983) *Code of Professional Practice*, United Kingdom Central Council for Nursing, Midwifery and Health Visiting (23 Portland Place, London W1N 3AF)

UN Convention (1991) *The Rights of the Child*, National Children's Bureau

Walklin, L. (1991) *The Assessment of Performance and Competence*, Cheltenham: Stanley Thornes

Working Together under the Children Act (1989) London: The Stationery Office

Young, P. (1985) *Mastering Social Welfare*, Basingstoke: Macmillan

Index